Foreword by
David Berenbaum
Renowned Affordable & Fair Housing Advocate

Unsheltered

None of Us Are Home
Until All of Us Are Home

Peggy Willms & Dennis Pitocco

Book Interior and E-book Design by Amit Dey

UNSHELTERED: None of Us Are Home Until All of Us Are Home
ISBN: 978-1-955668-68-2 (Paperback)
ISBN: 978-1-955668-69-9 (EBook)
Library of Congress Control Number: 2024913801

WELLNESS
BOOKS
AUTHENTIC ENDEAVORS
PUBLISHING

AuthenticEndeavorsPublishing.com

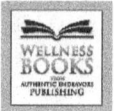

DISCLAIMER

"Unsheltered" is a compilation of personal stories, experiences, recollections, and perspectives contributed by various authors. The stories published in this book are the sole and individual expressions of each respective contributing author.

The contributing authors are solely responsible for the accuracy, authenticity, and ethical considerations pertaining to their individual contributions.

It is important to note that the perspectives and opinions expressed in this book do not necessarily reflect the views or opinions of the co-authors or the publisher. The co-authors have collaborated in the compilation and editing process, but their involvement is limited to facilitating the presentation of diverse perspectives on this topic.

The publisher has made reasonable efforts to ensure the accuracy and integrity of the content within the book, but does not assume responsibility for the individual viewpoints, opinions, or factual accuracy of each author's contribution. The stories presented are subjective and based on personal experiences.

Table of Contents

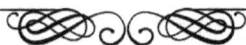

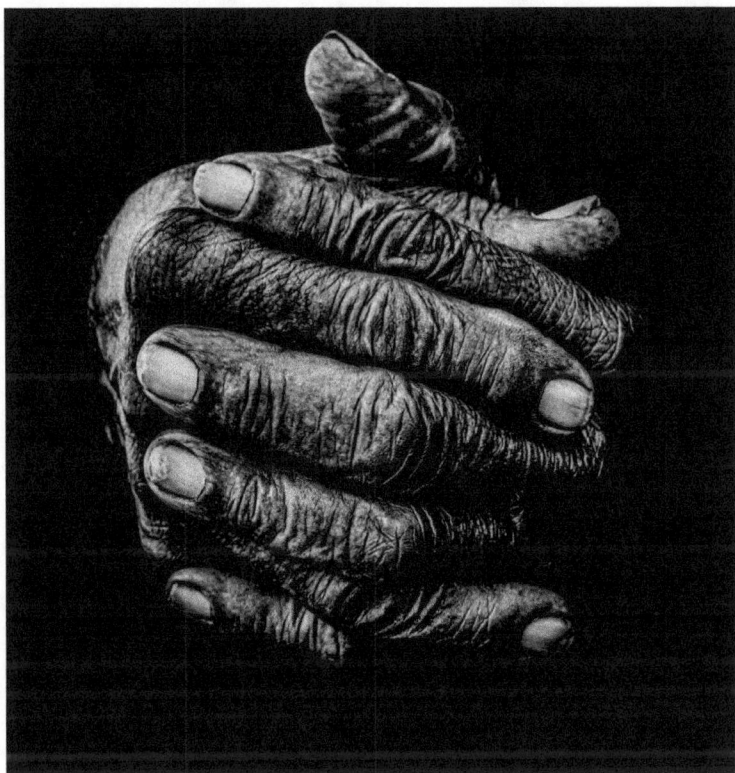

Dignity No Matter What: Collector Edition 2023
Renato Rampolla

Mario

Mario generously allowed me to capture a close-up photograph of his hands, showcasing his habitual resting posture. Remarkably, this image now graces the cover of "Unsheltered," a poignant book that delves into the complexities of homelessness.

Renato Rampolla

Acknowledgments

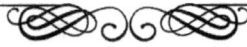

First and foremost, I thank our storytellers whose true, transparent, and authentic stories improve our knowledge, respect, and love for mankind. You have forever changed me.

To my Co-Author and great friend – the Batman to my Robin-Dennis Pitocco – I told you this journey was one I would only take if you walked along with me. You dove in head first. Somedays we laughed, cried, screamed, or all three, but we "soldiered on." I am grateful for you.

To David Berenbaum, who wrote our Foreword. Thank you for having the heart and courage to print your knowledge, experience, and views in this book. Your insight and passion give us a glimpse into your personal and professional behind-the-scenes work, which I greatly respect.

To Renato Rampolla and Sarah Harvey, photographers, and singer/songwriter Rocky Michaels, thank you for allowing your beautifully creative work be displayed on these pages.

Thank you to our publisher, Teresa Velardi and her team, who donated their time to this not-for-profit project. A special thank you to Susan Rooks, the Grammar Goddess. There were days I couldn't spell my name and you stood by me without judgement. To our Media Partners, thank for your passion in transmitting truths and helping us bring attention to such a global epidemic.

To my family and friends, thank you for allowing me the space and respect to write four books simultaneously. Your love is unwavering, and I love and thank you immensely.

Peggy Willms, Co-Author
CFT, SPN, CHLWC, author, host,
All Things Wellness, owner

*W*hat started out as a journey into the unknown evolved into not only a labor of love, but an extraordinary personal learning experience. I thought I understood what home-lessness meant. I thought gathering stories would be a straightforward experience. But from my first encounter with a man named "John" on the streets of Edinburgh, Scotland, to my conversations on the streets of Tampa Bay, this story gathering endeavor has positively changed me "for good."

This book would not have been possible without the incredible courage and resilience of the individuals who shared their stories with us. To each storyteller within who opened up about their experience of homelessness either directly or because of a friend or relative spent time on the streets, we are forever grateful. Your willingness to be vulnerable and give voice to realities that often go unseen was a profound gift. Thank you for trusting us with your truths.

To my kindred spirit, confidant, and Co-Author, Peggy Willms. Your inspiration sparked this journey. Your priceless wisdom of experience, candid insights, creativity, sense of humor in the midst of every challenge faced, and unwavering support has enriched every page. This work is a testament to your ability to gracefully lead with your heart. Thank you for being an exceptional collaborator and friend.

I also wish to extend my deepest gratitude to those who facilitated connections and created spaces where these narratives could be shared safely and without judgment. Your compassion and commitment to uplifting marginalized voices is simply inspiring.

To my friends and family who supported me through this project, providing encouragement when the weight of these stories became heavy to carry, thank you. Your empathy and care sustained me.

Finally, to every reader who picks up this book, I hope the stories within move you as they have moved me — instilling greater empathy, eroding stigmas, and inspiring action to build a more just and equitable society for all.

Dennis Pitocco, Co-Author
Chief ReImaginator, 360° Nation

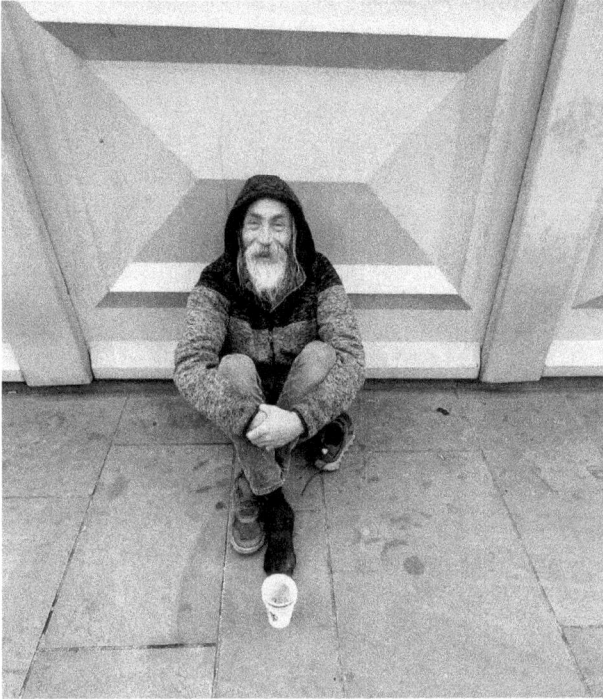

Dennis Pitocco, Photographer

"John"
Edinburgh, Scotland

Foreword

By David Berenbaum

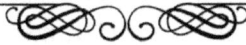

*W*e live in a world where we face numerous personal and community challenges that demand our attention. From the simple, such as what we should have for dinner or whether my paycheck cleared, to the complex, for example, global warming, COVID-19, or the focus of *Unsheltered*, the plight of the homeless worldwide.

The truth is that many societal issues we face can be solved, including ensuring everyone has an affordable and safe place to call home. If we open our hearts and minds to the issue, brush off the stereotypes that have misinformed our perceptions, and resolve to make a difference, we can ensure affordable housing for all. From a social, public policy, and even a theological perspective, we must embrace and acknowledge the critical importance of affirmatively furthering solutions for "unsheltered" people both around the world and across the street. Housing is critical to many other facets of life, including physical and mental health, access to employment, and financial wellbeing, among many others.

We invite you to consider the people, stories, and photographs in *Unsheltered* from a new perspective and to "see" the unhoused as people. Their life stories will surprise you with their candor, experiences, how they lost their housing, and how they confronted their challenges to enjoy a fresh start. We are humbled and appreciative of the "storytellers" who came forward to share their journeys and break down the stereotypes perpetuated over the years. This creates an opportunity for us to put a true face to the issue and pursue meaningful solutions at home and worldwide.

First, let's ground our discussion.

We will use the wording "unsheltered" and "unhoused" in the anthology series rather than the expression "homeless." This is not an exercise in political correctness but reflects the growing consensus of professionals, advocates, and practitioners worldwide[1] that the unsheltered are, in fact, our neighbors and live in the cities and communities that we all call home. This understanding is a critical first step to humanizing the issue and approaching the global crisis with empathy.

So, who are the unhoused or at risk of being unsheltered?

The answer is remarkably similar around the world.

They are people just like you and me. They are the elderly, young adults, and families with children. They are employees of big-box retailers who cannot afford the market value rent near their workplace and live out of their car. They are college students using their campus as a place to sleep and the gym to shower. They are seniors and older adults who cannot sustain their housing due to financial abuse, inadequate income, or prolonged hospitalization. They have served our nation. They are women and children who have experienced physical and/or sexual victimization. Many individuals have experienced or continue to experience emotional, physical, and mental health and substance abuse challenges. They are moms and dads, grandparents, people with disabilities, members of our faith communities who exist daily on their income, and most importantly, they are our neighbors.

In December of 2022, the United States Department of Housing and Urban Development issued the 2023 Annual Assessment Report, which provides estimates on the extent of this significant social issue in the United States. On a single night in 2023, roughly 653,100 people in the United States were unsheltered – a 12% increase, or about 706,590 more people than in 2022. Among people experiencing homelessness, 60% were staying in sheltered locations, while 40% were experiencing

---

[1] Is it OK to use the word 'homeless' – or should you say 'unhoused'? | Poverty | The Guardian

unsheltered homelessness in places not meant for human habitation. This January 2023 Point-in-Time (PIT) count is the highest number of people reported as being unhoused since reporting began in 2007.[2]

About three in every ten people experiencing homelessness (28%) did so as part of a family with children.

Most people experiencing homelessness were individuals, making up 72% of people experiencing homelessness. Between 2022 and 2023, the number of individuals experiencing unsheltered homelessness increased by 23,000 people, or 11%. The number of individuals experiencing sheltered homelessness increased by about 15,000, or 7%. Nearly 28% of people experiencing homelessness (186,100) were in families composed of at least one adult and one child. The number of families experiencing homelessness rose by 16% (more than 25,000 people) between 2022 and 2023, ending a downward trend that began in 2012. This increase in family homelessness was driven by a 17% increase (24,966 more people) in the number of families experiencing sheltered homelessness.[3]

In the United States, people who identify as Black, Latino, American Indian, Alaska Native, Pacific Islander, or Native Hawaiian continue to be overrepresented among the homeless population compared to the U.S. population. People who identify as Black, for example, represent 13% of the U.S. population but accounted for 37% of all people experiencing homelessness, and 50% of families experiencing homelessness in 2023 identified as Black. Nearly one-third of all people experiencing homelessness identified as Hispanic or Latino. People identifying as Hispanic or Latino increased by 28% (39,106 people) between 2022 and 2023, making up 55% of the total increase in people experiencing homelessness. People who identify as Asian or

[2] 2023 AHAR: Part 1 - PIT Estimates of Homelessness in the U.S. | HUD USER
[3] The 2023 Annual Homelessness Assessment Report (AHAR to Congress) Part 1: Point-In-Time Estimates of Homelessness, December 2023 (huduser.gov)

Asian American experienced the greatest percentage increase among all people experiencing homelessness, representing a 40% increase (3,313 more people) between 2022 and 2023. American Indian, Alaska Native, or Indigenous populations also experienced a large percentage increase in both sheltered and unsheltered experiences of individual homelessness between 2022 and 2023, both of which rose by 18-19% (or 2,860 people total).[4]

Between 2022 and 2023, the number of unaccompanied youth increased by 15% (4,613 more youths). According to the report, more than 98,000 people experiencing homelessness were aged 55 to 64, and nearly 39,700 people were over age 64. Nearly half of adults of age 55 and older experiencing homelessness were experiencing unsheltered homelessness in places not meant for human habitation. In 2023, 35,574 veterans were experiencing homelessness, marking a 7% increase (2,445 more veterans) between 2023 and 2023. Despite increases in veteran homelessness between 2022 and 2023, the number of veterans experiencing homelessness is 52% lower than it was in 2009.[5] The Housing First model – which is used by the U.S. Department of Veterans Affairs (VA) in its two largest homelessness programs – has been instrumental in reducing veteran homelessness by more than 55 percent over the past decade.[6] In 2021, 72% of veterans experiencing sheltered homelessness had a disability.[7]

In my experience, most individuals and families I have advocated for or provided fair housing and housing counseling services to are only one paycheck away from losing their homes[8]. Something as minor as an

---

[4] The 2023 Annual Homelessness Assessment Report (AHAR to Congress) Part 1: Point-In-Time Estimates of Homelessness, December 2023 (huduser.gov)
[5] The 2023 Annual Homelessness Assessment Report (AHAR to Congress) Part 1: Point-In-Time Estimates of Homelessness, December 2023 (huduser.gov)
[6] New Data Shows 11% Decline in Veteran Homelessness Since 2020 – the Biggest Drop in More Than 5 Years | HUD.gov / U.S. Department of Housing and Urban Development (HUD)
[7] The 2023 Annual Homelessness Assessment Report (AHAR to Congress) Part 1: Point-In-Time Estimates of Homelessness, December 2023 (huduser.gov)
[8] Charles Schwab – Logica Research

emergency room visit or an unexpected car expense could take three out of five employees from making ends meet to a catastrophe[9]. Imagine the impact of losing your job, the loss of a spouse, or any other life-changing event on your personal finances. Financial insecurity and the shortage of affordable housing for all income groups are substantial domestic and global challenges.

Things have only worsened since the pandemic, with three times as many people having less savings for a rainy day today.[10] Do you know someone who is "doubled-up" or "couch surfing" because they cannot afford a place of their own? I am sure you do. They are also considered unsheltered, though not captured in the HUD National Homeless Assessment Report data I cited earlier. Besides elders struggling to age in place on a fixed income, many older Americans living on a fixed income in Florida, California, Colorado, Hawaii, and Louisiana who could not afford to maintain their homeowner's insurance allowed it to lapse. Unfortunately, they are unsheltered and have been displaced from their "forever" homes due to severe hurricanes, fires, floods, and other natural disasters. Sadly, older Americans who need affordable housing are arguably the fastest-growing group of the unhoused.

Globally, underlying issues and causation of displacement are very similar to those in the United States.

However, although it is commonly known and accepted that there are millions of unhoused people worldwide, it is challenging to quantify the exact number with any degree of accuracy due to the absence of data.[11] The United Nations[12] estimates that approximately 1.6 billion people reside in poor housing worldwide, with around 15 million being forcibly

---

[9] 63% of workers are unable to pay a $500 emergency expense: survey (cnbc.com)

[10] https://www.bankrate.com/banking/savings/emergency-savings-survey-2020/

[11] Homelessness by Country 2023 (worldpopulationreview.com)

[12] United Nations Secretariat – Multilateral from USA – Conflict, Disaster Reduction, Education, Health, Humanitarian Aid & Emergency, Security sectors – Development Aid

evicted each year.[13] As inflation increases globally, so does rent, making this statistic even more troubling.

Examples from across the globe show the complexity of addressing housing crises, even when housing is declared a human right. For example, natural disasters and conflicts cause people to lose their homes and seek new shelter. The worldwide shortage of safe and affordable housing is another major cause. Again, like in the United States, many people in other industrialized nations are unable to pay their rent or mortgage due to unemployment, which can be caused by an economic crisis, the pandemic, or physical or mental issues. Numerous factors, many of which are also interconnected with health, nutrition, and global warming, contribute to the phenomenon. And while the United Nations and several nations have proclaimed that access to affordable housing is a human right, we have a long way to go before achieving this ambitious goal.

In fact, an affordable and safe place to call home was first recognized as a human right in the 1948 Universal Declaration of Human Rights[14]. It has since been reaffirmed in many international treaties, resolutions, and declarations[15]. Both globally and in the United States, the framing of housing as a human right continues to garner significant policy and public attention.[16] However, the shortage of affordable housing stubbornly persists.

The United Nations, in its "Special Rapporteur on Homelessness and Human Rights," reports that housing the unsheltered has emerged as a global human rights issue and that the unhoused are often stigmatized, addressed with criminalization, violence, and aggressive policies that violate, rather than safeguard, the rights of the persons involved.[17]

Further, regardless of resources in the nation involved, the unhoused are often discriminated against based on their housing status or due to

---

[13] Everyone included – how to end homelessness | United Nations
[14] Universal Declaration of Human Rights | OHCHR
[15] https://housingmatters.urban.org/articles/naming-housing-human-right-first-step-solving-housing-crisis
[16] 01-06_Housing-Human-Right.pdf (nlihc.org)
[17] Homelessness and human rights | OHCHR

their lack of official address, affecting their political, economic, and social rights, such as their right to participate in elections, their right to work, or their right to access certain social benefits. The Special Rapporteur pragmatically acknowledges the complexity of this social issue and reaffirms the need for every nation to make reasonable efforts to guarantee access to safe, affordable, and adequate housing as a core human rights issue.

In the United States, this is often demonstrated by source of income discrimination against the unhoused who receive rental subsidy support through federal, state, or local public sector programs, such as the United States Department of Housing & Urban Development Section Eight Rental Subsidy Voucher program or related Continuum of Care programs. Even though these programs will pay for a substantial portion of a qualified tenant's low-to-moderate consumer rent, many landlords refuse to accept the subsidy. Fair housing and affordable housing advocates view this refusal as a pretext for housing discrimination; notably, many local jurisdictions are now passing legislation to prevent source-of-income discrimination.

The unhoused are often categorized into three groups − the chronic, episodic, and transitional homeless. For the unhoused, these impersonal and "clinical" terms belie the human cost and emotional and financial distress that so many at-risk and unhoused individuals face. Even though an unprecedented number of market-rate apartments have been built over the past decade, the rent for these new units is out of reach. Ironically, many of these upscale and luxury units are sitting unrented in markets across the nation, with a significant need for affordable rental units demonstrating the need for inclusive zoning ordinances smart growth.

Inflation has also chipped away for those on fixed incomes, creating a daily reality where low- to moderate-income households do not have enough income to pay for necessities such as food, clothing, transportation, and a place to call home. Significantly, the cost of and access to health care compounds the situation and creates the perfect storm, leading to eviction or foreclosure.

While many communities represent – may I say pretend – they don't have a "homeless issue," ignore the unhoused, or even try to make these residents go away, the reality is that denial is not a solution, and this is simply a group of people without homes who quietly live among us. Many don't want you to know they don't have a roof over their heads for fear of how they will be treated.

Tent cities have emerged in metropolitan areas across the globe because of poverty, political and economic challenges, war, natural and manmade disasters, and so many other societal issues. And while we can close our eyes and walk or drive by someone who is unsheltered on the street, many choose to ignore the issue or even be cruel. Neither approach does anything or solves the issue. But together, we can change this paradigm. To quote Dr. Martin Luther King, Jr., "We all came in on different ships, but we're in the same boat now."

As you turn the pages of this book, I urge you to imagine yourself walking in the shoes of the people sharing their experiences and stories with you. Imagine what your day would be like, how others would perceive you, and what services and programs you would require. Could you afford housing in your community? What do you see in the eyes of those who have been photographed? Do you know what living in a shelter is like? Do people choose to be homeless or even live on the street? Who will be in your corner and help you have a fresh start? It's time for the unsheltered stories to be told by them and by all of us who can bring our collective talent and voices to the issue.

**There are many solutions that one can support
to help the unhoused, fight poverty,
and provide more affordable housing.**

We hope that the personal stories, journeys, and "truths" shared through the interviews, essays, and photography in *Unsheltered: Voices from the Street* will surprise you and eloquently focus your attention on the human condition and plight of the unsheltered. The next time you meet someone who is unhoused, take the time to speak with that person if you feel comfortable. I hope that it will be a joy for each of you. Then, please consider getting involved with countless not-for-profit and non-governmental organizations (NGOs) worldwide, partnering with the public and private sectors to make a difference. Some of the agencies' work is also highlighted in *Unsheltered*.

Unsheltered is a labor of love to put a face to the issue, share the stories of those who have fallen on hard times, who are unhoused or at risk of becoming unsheltered, and expand our understanding of the need for smart growth that celebrates solutions, compassion, and the availability of social services and housing. Everyone who is part of this project is volunteering their time, talent, and passion to make a difference and be a voice for change. I hope you will be moved after reading the real-life stories and seeing the powerful photography featured in *Unsheltered*. More importantly, we hope that you will join us in supporting our neighbors in need.

None of us are home until all of us are home.

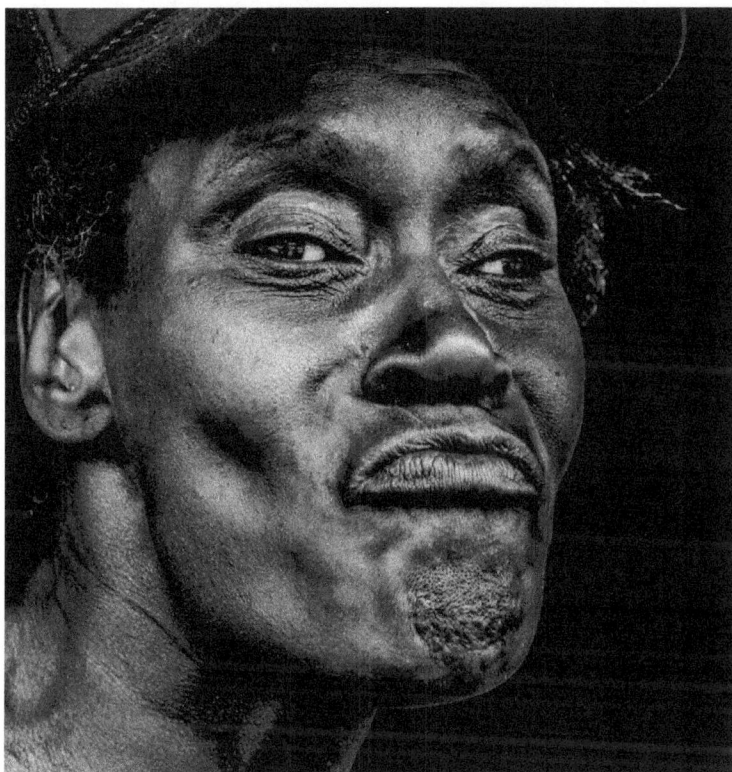

Dignity No Matter What: Collector Edition 2023
Renato Rampolla

Sylvia

It was a brisk morning, and all she asked for was a cup of coffee. I bought her one, and she was so grateful you would have thought I bought her a diamond watch. Sylvia has good days and bad, more than that, she has days when she really isn't herself and she gets angry. Today, she was feeling good.

Preface

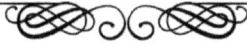

*H*omelessness has long been one of the most vexing and persistent social challenges facing societies around the world. While often rendered invisible by the crowds and commotion of urban life, the harsh reality is that on any given night, millions of men, women, and children worldwide struggle without a safe, permanent place to call home. Exposed to the elements, hunger, violence, and a continual denial of basic human dignity, those experiencing homelessness confront unimaginable hardship, trauma, and dehumanization.

What sets this book apart is our intentional groundbreaking emphasis on elevating the authentic voices and first-hand perspectives of those who have lived through the homelessness crisis. At its core, this is an experiential journey that takes you to the streets and shelters through raw, powerful narratives from people still trapped in the cycle of housing insecurity as well as the illuminating voices of those who have managed to transition out of homelessness against all odds. By sharing their intimate, heartrending stories and hard-earned insights, this book puts a human face on the often, dehumanizing experience of life without shelter.

This book also critically captures the perspectives and testimonies of those who have been profoundly impacted by having family or friends living without stable housing. Their stories shed light on the profound ripple effects that homelessness has on surrounding communities and personal relationships when a parent, child, sibling, or loved one falls into this darkest of circumstances. By including this diversity of perspectives from varied vantage points, a truly multidimensional picture of the homelessness crisis emerges in these pages.

These visceral first-hand accounts from varied lived experiences align with our objective, that is; to raise widespread awareness by dispelling the dangerous myths, assumptions, and dehumanizing stereotypes that too often shape public perception. This book also strives to issue an impassioned call to action on solving this humanitarian crisis that haunts cities and communities in every corner of the world.

Over the following chapters, you'll gain a comprehensive, unflinching exploration of just who experiences homelessness and why. It delves unflinchingly into the complex web of societal factors that lead to housing insecurity – from a lack of affordable housing stock, stagnant wages, and generational poverty to systemic problems like mental illness, substance abuse, domestic violence, and individual trauma that remain unresolved and untreated. Along the way, we do not shy away from difficult truths, spotlighting the unique challenges and vulnerabilities faced by specific populations like homeless families with children, and at-risk veterans.

Ultimately, this book makes the powerful case that homelessness is not just a crisis impacting those living without shelter. Its effects intimately shape the public spaces of our cities, strain public resources like emergency rooms and correctional facilities, fuel neighborhood tensions and "not in my backyard" attitudes and weigh heavily on the national conscience about whether we are truly living up to our ideals as a just, equitable, and compassionate society.

While the path to implementing true solutions is extraordinarily complex from a policy and resource perspective, overcoming homelessness must be viewed as a moral and ethical imperative for any society that values human rights, equality of opportunity, the full realization of human potential, and the preservation of fundamental human dignity for all people.

By amplifying the long-marginalized voices of those who have experienced homelessness firsthand, as well as those deeply and personally impacted by this crisis, our profound hope is that this book can foster greater understanding, empathy, and an unwavering commitment to sustainable and proven solutions. We hope readers will be inspired to get educated, get involved through advocacy or direct service, and get behind efforts to finally make transformative progress against one of our greatest societal ills.

For until this challenge is overcome through a holistic, compassionate, and human-centered approach, we cannot honestly call ourselves a just, equitable society that protects and uplifts the most vulnerable among us. The struggle of our homeless neighbors, family members, and fellow human beings must be a struggle that weighs upon all of our consciences. We can and must do better as a civilization to solve this moral crisis in our midst. The time is long overdue to change the narrative by understanding what it's really like to live on the street – and to bring care and compassion to those who walk among us day in and out who seek not only food, water, and shelter, but who seek to escape the soul-crunching impact of invisibility.

Introduction

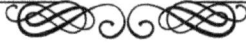

If you're expecting fresh insights into trends, statistics, government studies, and bureaucratic policy regurgitation, you've simply picked up the wrong book. Why? Because our unwavering objective from day one has been to cut through the crap and repetitive baloney by capturing unvarnished perspectives from those who truly know what it's like to live on the streets because they live there, today or they once lived there, and have the courage to share their stories. Period.

And unlike virtually all other books focused on homelessness, we didn't immerse ourselves in mind-numbing academic research, nor did we hide behind the scenes hoping for folks to come forward. We went to them. We went to the streets. We sat with them, spoke with them, and gave them something they seek beyond food, water, and shelter. We gave them the elusive visibility they so dearly long for.

What readers can expect from this book is an immersive exploration of homelessness, unlike any other work on the subject. Through searing first-person testimony and frontline insights, these pages will shatter misconceptions and lay bare the harsh realities of one of society's most devastating humanitarian crises in utterly unflinching terms. The stories and perspectives enclosed within will leave an indelible mark on the reader's conscience.

The visceral, haunting accounts from those whose lives have been upended by homelessness will inspire a complex mix of powerful emotions. There will be rage – rage at the dehumanizing injustice, indignity, and unconscionable suffering that hundreds of thousands of our fellow human beings are forced to endure each day and night while struggling to survive in a perpetual state of housing insecurity and destitution. Raw anger will swell at the individual and systemic failings that have allowed such cruelty and deprivation to persist.

At the same time, these stories will cultivate profound admiration, even awe, at the resilience, courage, creativity, and perseverance required to endure the physical, psychological, and spiritual gauntlet of homelessness. To maintain one's basic human dignity and sense of selfhood while routinely being stripped of privacy, security, social ties, purpose, and fundamental rights is an act of unparalleled strength. Readers will feel humbled and inspired by those who have walked this arduous path mere steps away from them, yet worlds apart.

There will be abundant doubt, second-guessing and self-reflection catalyzed within readers' psyches as they are brought face-to-face with the human face of the crisis and the myriad systemic factors that perpetuate it. Long-held preconceptions and prejudices about the perceived "reasons" and "choices" behind homelessness will be laid bare as the myths and dehumanizing stereotypes they truly are. Readers will be forced to confront their own complacency, privilege, and complicity in allowing such dehumanizing conditions and disparities to persist.

And ultimately, this reckoning with the sheer scale, trauma, and societal rot that the crisis represents will leave readers with an abiding sense of sorrow and shame – sorrow for the countless human potentials reduced to mere survival, and shame that such degrading suffering is allowed to fester in even the wealthiest, most resource-rich nation on earth and beyond. How can such indignity be permitted to persist in a society that purports to value human rights, human dignity, equality, justice, and basic decency above all else?

However, this book does not wallow in hopelessness, nor apportion blame as an end unto itself. For woven between the heart-rending accounts of homelessness are the stories of those who have chosen a different path – the tenacious advocates, frontline outreach workers, shelter operators, policy reformers, and multitudes of compassionate individuals who have dedicated their lives and earnest efforts to easing suffering and charting a way out of this moral morass. Their wisdom, innovative spirit, empathy, and abiding faith in human potential will shine through as beacons of hope even in the darkest chapters

Readers will draw strength, purpose and a revitalized sense of civic obligation from these inspiring accounts of those selflessly fighting against injustice and for the universal human right of housing. The perseverance and profound loving-kindness of these modern-day heroes and trailblazers will serve as a clarion call for each and every reader to transcend apathy, despair and diffusion of responsibility. For in bearing unflinching witness to the scale and depravity of the crisis laid bare, one cannot resist the moral duty to get off the sidelines and into the struggle to change this inexcusable status quo.

Indeed, this book's most vital contribution will be serving as the spark to reawaken individual and collective consciousness. By peeling away the peculiar willful ignorance so many have embraced around homelessness and shining an unfiltered spotlight through a rich tapestry of first-hand perspectives, apathy will become untenable. The blinders will be removed, and the full scope of this moral crisis impacting millions will finally be rendered inescapable – but not as a source of resignation or despair.

Rather, this unvarnished examination of the homelessness crisis is intended as a profound call to action, a permanent awakening of the conscience, and a challenge to one's civic values, ethics and basic humanity. For in the end, readers will be left with an unshakable understanding – a visceral emotional knowledge etched upon their very souls – that homelessness is not just a blight upon those experiencing it directly. Its very existence as a societal scourge marks an injurious blight upon us all.

The struggle of our homeless neighbors, family members, and fellow human beings cast into the cruelties of housing insecurity must become a struggle that weighs upon all of our individual consciences. We cannot pay lip service to concepts of compassion, justice and human flourishing while simultaneously averting our gaze from such lacerating injustice. We cannot honestly call ourselves an ethical, equitable, or truly advanced civilization until this moral crisis is resolved in a holistic, empathetic, and human-centered manner that permanently upholds the universal human right to safe, secure shelter with access to supportive services.

By bearing unsparing witness through these pages, this book aims to spark a true nationwide – and worldwide – reawakening and movement to achieve that aim. It implores all who experience its testimony and insights to not retreat into despair or diffusion of responsibility, but rather burn with "a fierce urgency of now" and channel that emotional gravity into sustained, concrete action. For the struggle of our homeless neighbors must become all of our struggles, their trauma, our trauma, their indignity, our shared indignity. Only through such an elevated consciousness and united front can we hope to forge a truly just society worthy of its highest ideals.

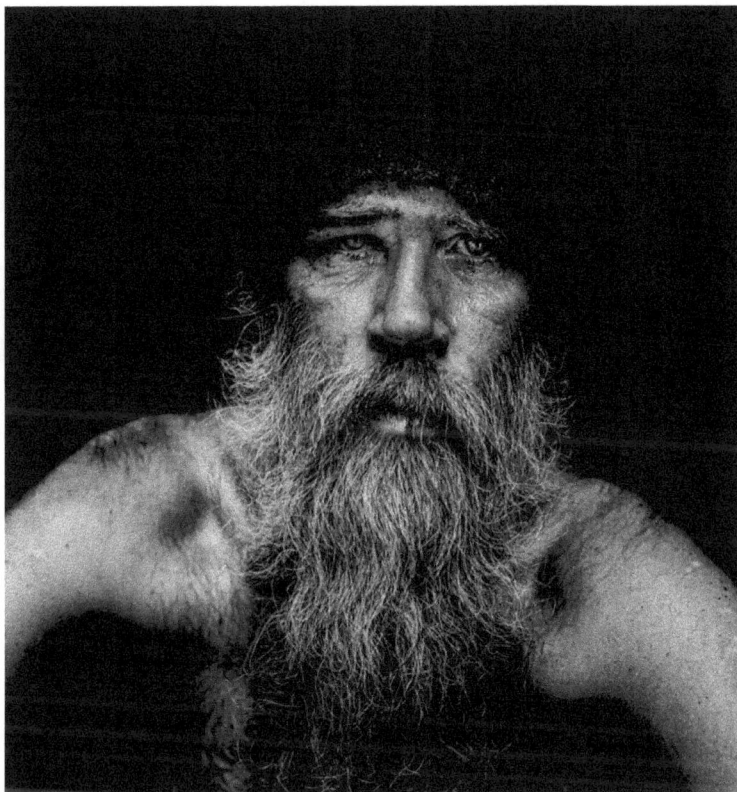

Dignity No Matter What: Collector Edition 2023
Renato Rampolla

Daniel

I noticed him staggering on the sidewalk in the summer heat. His sneakers were untied and he wore no shirt. I could easily count each of his ribs through his pale skin. He is tall, so tall that he towered over most people he passed. I followed him to the safe place he had made with his blankets in the portico of a vacant building.

He smiled when I asked his name. Daniel, he said. I gave him a bottle of water and sat down with him. He smelled of sweat, beer, and urine. We talked a while as I took several pictures.

After a few minutes, tears appeared in his eyes as he said, "I appreciate that you see me...who I am, not how I look now. Thanks, man."

His mouth opened as if he were going to say something else, but he didn't. He just gazed right into my eyes as if he were searching for something, perhaps an answer, I don't know. He wept and I put my hand on his shoulder.

"Of course, Daniel, but no need to thank me for that. Where do you go from here?"

He stared right through me and said nothing. There was no hope in his eyes, and I felt a deep sense of hollowness.

Focusing my lens on people who are destitute can be taxing as listening to their stories and situations is a lot to bear. However, many of these people have a certain fortitude, beauty and strength that I admire.

This is my encounter with Daniel almost five years ago. Daniel's appreciation of me seeing him as a man and not a label was one of the main reasons I decided I needed to make the book.

I met Daniel in Soho, NY. I have been back several times over the years and have not seen him again.

I See You

By Peggy Willms

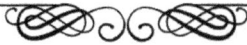

$\mathcal{J}$ rom Mount Everest's peaks to the Dead Sea's basins, there is still not enough distance to express the vast lessons I have experienced while on the journey to share stories from those unfortunately unsheltered or homeless.

For the last three years, my purpose has been to be the vessel to tell and share stories, whether in print or on air. I believe harboring our stories and experiences is a disservice to the world. God sparked me with the concept of writing a compilation book of those unsheltered after attending a get-together with my Co-Author, Dennis Pitocco, who, frankly, may have initially thought I was biting off a rather large chew. And I was. Dennis had worked with this population, and I had written three compilation books—a great fit. After one meeting, I was honored when he said yes.

I was assured he was the best partner for me to change the narrative and perceptions of those not "living on the streets." We were on the same page, metaphorically and quite literally. For Dennis, it was a fantastic concept, but how could we honor these potential contributing authors, how would we gather stories safely, and would it make a difference in the long run? I told him I wanted the profits to go back into the communities that serve this population, and frankly, he needed to hang on because I believed in us as a team. I wanted no money and knew he needed to be my partner, or I wouldn't do it. The rest is history.

And here we are with you.

Our mission was to rally our collective talent and resources to materially amplify the voices and visibility of the unsheltered population while breaking down the stigma associated with homelessness. We listen, gather, and share their stories. We change the world by changing the narrative, one person, one story, one day at a time.

We felt it's time to open our minds and our hearts by doing MORE and doing BETTER, as together, we educate, raise awareness of, and dismantle the misconceptions about the many misunderstood souls living on the street, empowering each of us—individually and collectively—to create change for good.

From David's Foreword, Renato's photo submissions, Rocky's anthem, the publishing team (including editors, formatter, and illustrator), to creating contracts, a website landing page, marketing, and more...we soldiered on day after day for 15 months. I pray that you hold these stories as dear to your heart and with respect as this whole team has.

I have never been exposed to someone who is homeless, though I have worked with a few who "have been." Along the way in gathering these stories, I have experienced a gamut of emotions: anger, love, and confusion while working with the contributing authors to a level of disgust, confusion, and sheer embarrassment as to who should be stepping up to the plate to help this population and design real solutions. The latter has put me in a few precarious positions, yet I still stand by my actions and reactions.

You, too, will experience an emotional journey as you proceed through the fantastic stories of courage, excitement, and sheer fear. I shed many tears, and, in some cases, I had to stop editing many stories midway before needing a deep breath, tissue, or to walk away for a bit. Even typing this stirs mixed emotions. I cannot believe how the whole team, including our contributing authors, came together to accomplish such a feat. By reading these stories, you may just put on their shoes or lack thereof, and you may just learn to love them as I have.

We worked with every one of the contributing authors in this book. We worked diligently to place their precious words on the pages you see before you.. These are their stories, NOT ours. They have permitted us to publicize their experiences, and many stated the cathartic writing process has been life-changing. Most were ecstatic that we cared that we would listen. Some stories rolled in on paper and others in interviews.

Some contributors are authors, singers, lawyers, teenagers, parents, etc. They are from around the world on nearly every continent. You may or may not know, but they are your friends, family members, co-workers, and neighbors. They are us!

We met storytellers virtually and in person and spoke on the phone. Even "Hollywood" called us to do a documentary, but we turned them down. Some storytellers are public about their experience, and some are still in physical "hiding." We talked to those who find being "unsheltered" safer than living in their own home. That statement flowed most often from the mouths of babes: teenagers "on the run." We spoke with those escaping domestic violence, those who lost jobs, and frankly, a few who have chosen to live on the streets as they seek the simplicity and self-control their current environment offers.

The most shocking experience I had was all but one of the nonprofits we approached either didn't return our calls or emails, or they were initially ecstatic we asked them to be involved; however, we never heard from them again. That is an example of why my emotions of disgust, confusion, and sheer embarrassment come into play. I was and am still livid.

How will we understand how to help and contribute to changing the narrative of those unfortunate if the exact people who serve the warm meals and hand out blankets will not meet with us? Why? What is the secret? Are you too busy? Do you want help from those of us trying to make a difference in these lives? Perhaps you can enlighten me as to the "real" reasons. Is it fear, distrust, or lack of desire?

I sought out the who, what, where, when, why, and how. I use the *6Ws of Wellness* in my practice, so I thought the process would be fitting for this journey as well. I needed answers. And foolishly, I thought we would receive most of the stories through the homeless shelters and soup kitchens. They knew the population, and indeed, they would offer us a safe environment in which to gather them! No! This was one of my greatest disappointments.

About two stories in, I became overwhelmed with who was stepping up currently and who would be a part of the solution moving forward. Who is willing to learn more about the 6Ws of homelessness by reading a book such as this, watching a video, or visiting a shelter themselves? I know you are interested in the subject or your eyes would not be scanning these pages. I have hope for the humans around the globe. I believe in one love and that we can all, collectively, make this world a better place.

I remain steadfast in enhancing my knowledge and walking the talk. After all, statistics show that we are all just a few paychecks away from not having a roof over our head and looking for a swig of water and a blanket to shed off the brisk night.

I am sparked by what I learned from the brilliant souls willing to tell their stories—those who shared their words with us and now with you.

This journey has been one of the most emotional yet rewarding experiences in my life.

I can guarantee you a few things. I WILL offer a bottle of water or energy bar to someone struggling to get their next meal. I WILL continue to seek knowledge and under-standing. I WILL listen more. And I WILL SEE them. They are us, and one person at a time does and WILL make a difference in seeking solutions to leave this world happier and healthier than we found it.

Gimme Shelter:
What's It Really Like To Be Homeless?

By Dennis Pitocco

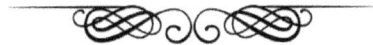

*How we walk with the broken speaks
louder than how we sit with the great.*

Bill Bennot

A weathered man, his face etched with the lines of hardship, sits hunched on a park bench. His worn coat, once vibrant, has faded to a dull grey, its threadbare seams struggling to hold it together. A weathered backpack, its straps frayed and patched, rests beside him, its contents a mystery of forgotten possessions and survival necessities. Once bright and full of life, his eyes now hold a deep weariness, yet a glimmer of defiance shines through. His gaze, fixed on the distant horizon, seems to carry the weight of countless stories, each a testament to the resilience of the human spirit in the face of adversity.

A weathered woman, her skin etched with a map of life's trials, sits huddled on a cold, concrete ledge. Her worn shawl, once a vibrant patchwork of colors, has faded to a drab tapestry of browns and greys, barely shielding her from the biting wind. A battered suitcase, its once proud leather now cracked and peeling, rests beside her, a repository of memories and forgotten dreams. Once filled with fire and spirit, her eyes now hold a quiet acceptance, reflecting the wisdom gleaned from years spent under the unforgiving sky. Her gaze, fixed on the bustling street below, seems to pierce the veil of anonymity, offering a glimpse into a soul that has weathered countless storms.

A family huddles together on another corner, seeking solace in their shared struggle. A young child, oblivious to the harsh realities of their situation, sleeps peacefully in his mother's arms. His innocent face, untouched by the world's harshness, offers a fleeting glimpse of hope and resilience. His parents, their faces etched with worry and exhaustion, shield their children from the harsh realities surrounding them, their love offering a temporary haven in a world that often seems unforgiving.

Down the road a bit, a group of teenagers huddle together, their laughter echoing through the stark emptiness of the abandoned building. Their faces, still bearing traces of childhood innocence, are hardened by the harsh realities of their situation. Their clothes, a mismatched collection of hand-me-downs and discarded garments, speak of a life lived on the margins of society. Yet, their laughter is a defiant challenge to their circumstances, a testament to the enduring power of human resilience.

These are just a few glimpses into the lives of those who live on the streets across the USA and across the world, each one a unique story of resilience and hardship. Beyond the labels of "homeless" or "vagrant," they are individuals with hopes and dreams, just like you and me. They deserve to be seen and heard, not as a problem to be solved, but as fellow human beings deserving of our compassion and understanding.

In the hustle and bustle of everyday life, we often pass by individuals whose struggles go unseen, unheard, and unacknowledged. These are the invisible homeless, those who navigate the complexities of life without the basic security of a roof over their heads. They may couch surf, sleep in cars, or find temporary shelter wherever they can. Unlike the more visible homeless population, they blend into the background, hidden from plain sight. But their invisibility does not diminish their humanity or struggles. To truly address the issue of homelessness, we must first cast light on their plight.

Walking With the Broken

Not long ago, I took to the streets of Tampa to "walk with the broken," seeking real voices from real people living on the street. How better to understand their dilemma than to listen to what they had to say about what it's really like to be homeless? As is the case in most cities, it's no secret where the homeless congregate—often where food is made available. Hence, my journey took me to the vicinity of a well-known food pantry on the "other" side of Tampa—the side where poverty is entrenched.

Having parked not far away, I approached the pantry intending to engage with each downtrodden soul I encountered. Little did I know that a more fruitful opportunity awaited as I noticed a small group of people beginning to gather just outside, waiting for the pantry doors to open for breakfast in less than an hour. Rather than single out each person gathered (my original plan), I simply stood alongside them all, hoping for an opportunity to chat.

And that's when I met Andrew, who, much to my surprise, walked up to me, reached out with a handshake, and a friendly "good morning." I responded in kind, with eye contact, introducing myself and asking his name, casually mentioning that I was doing research for a book intended to explain to the world what it was really like to be homeless through the eyes of those actually living on the street. "What's it like?" he questioned, then continued to share his perspectives. Before he finished his first sentence, I apologized for interrupting while gaining his permission to turn on my recorder, and then I stepped back to listen to every word.

And that's when the magic happened. As other people waited for the doors to open, they randomly joined the discussion, including Sally, Andrea, Tametta, Richard, Pete and Denzel. The conversation flowed, each playing off the other without skipping a beat until we were abruptly (and unfortunately) interrupted by the pantry doors swinging open, signaling "time for breakfast." While I was disappointed by the swift end of our group exchange, I understood how important it was for everyone to get a place in line for what might be their only meal that day.

An amazing encounter and, indeed, another learning experience for me—all because I was lucky enough to engage with the homeless on their terms and on their turf. And although (despite my original intentions) the only things I actually donated that morning were eye contact, visibility, and listening, their appreciative responses were both humbling and overwhelming. So, starting with Michael, I now share their candid, vulnerable, graphic, authentic, sobering, gut-wrenching answers to my question, "What's it REALLY like to be homeless?"

Andrew

"What's it like? People spit on you, kick you, beat you up, almost killed me once, steal your (empty) wallet, laugh at you, give you dirty looks, and most people judge you, call you names, and refer to you as homeless without understanding who you really are. It can be painful, scary, depressing, lonely, traumatic, exhausting, tragic, and cruel. My sadness is getting worse every day, and I'm considering taking my own life. My many disabilities make it challenging for me to work. Homelessness is by no means a good thing. It is physically, mentally, and spiritually torturous. In my experience, at least, it slowly kills you. Who, though, is going to miss me? Most of the time, I am invisible. It's just fatal to be homeless."

Sally

"I know in my heart that no one should be homeless. There are a lot of lies and misunderstandings about us homeless people, like the reason our families will not take us in—we are bad people, drug addicts, mentally ill, illiterate, have criminal records, don't want to work, or are just plain awful. A terminal illness is not as bad as homelessness or losing all the people you care about. Even though I've learned how to handle my issues, I frequently think that living when you're constantly this poor is not worth it. According to some, money isn't everything, but they haven't woken up on back-to-back birthdays and holidays, sweating in the suffocating humidity on the streets in too-small clothes, wearing broken shoes, with painful cavities, body aches, or insect bites. It's just terrible."

Andrea

"When you are on and off homeless, as I have been for the majority of my life, you are able to relate to other homeless people far more than you do to those who aren't on the street. We are just like everyone else. Our experiences are different from one another. If you aren't living on the street, you wouldn't understand anything if you listened to a normal conversation between us. We constantly discuss money above all else. If somebody hears of a church that paid someone's storage bill, gave them a gift card, or provided a motel voucher, these will be hot topics on our grapevine, and this stuff travels fast, like finding out about a coffee shop where you can sit without having to buy anything. Being homeless means that you can always count on other homeless people to relate to and understand what you are talking about. It's like we're on shared ground. It feels like we are separated from non-homeless people by an invisible wall. It resembles shop talk between you and your colleagues. If you're not homeless, you just don't get it."

Tametta

"I ain't never been homeless before now, but some unfortunate incidents in my life, including losing my job, bankruptcy, having a fire in my house, and having my car stolen, have led me to this situation. My fiancé and I are spending the night in a tent in a park not far from here and are having a hard time getting by. My kin have departed. My fiancé's family won't assist us. Everyone in our family and circle of friends has abandoned us. So, I would advise against expecting anyone to rescue or assist you when you live here on the street. Gain some basic skills and check around your neighborhood for odd jobs. Once you have a car, your chances of finding work increase."

Anonymous

"I was so scared the first night I was on the street a while ago. It's not the same as camping. I was worried about the weather and felt really vulnerable, always looking behind me and around me as I walked the streets. After a few days, I calmed down a bit because I found a few "hidden spots" to sleep in. After that, it was more about being able to find food pantries, blankets, toiletries and keeping myself safe day and night. I would rather trust my own abilities than depend on anybody else. Maintaining my hygiene and doing my laundry so that I can hunt for a job is the hardest thing.

I'm a little different from most homeless people I know who have given up looking because I haven't given up yet. My problem is you gotta have an address and phone number for employment applications. If your contact information is a charity, very few respectable jobs will take you seriously.

It's really hard to be on the streets and get ready for work every morning after I found a job after a month. It was a real balancing act, the two weeks between getting hired and getting my first paycheck. When I was younger and more confident, I could slip into various public locations to freshen up and spend a few hours indoors during the evening, but I'm sure security is much tighter these days."

Richard

"Being homeless isn't just about not having a home. It's not knowing how or when things will ever get better. It's being told repeatedly that you don't matter. That you're no one of consequence. You don't deserve help because you're not "special" enough. It's realizing you don't have what it takes to escape your situation. It's not knowing when, where, or if you'll get food again. It's realizing that you might have to look in a trash can for food if you do want to eat. Even though I have never used drugs in my life, everyone thinks I am a drug addict. Being homeless to me means you don't have anywhere to go and no family or friends to support you. Hopelessness is really what homelessness is."

Anonymous

"I had to get away fast from a very dangerous man, not even a romantic partner. Just a crazy psychopath I'd dated for a little while. Before assaulting me and imprisoning me in his house for ninety-two days, he had been stalking me for almost two years, leaving me with a traumatic brain injury, severe PTSD, and a broken knee.

I left my house, my friends, my family, and my entire life behind to move a thousand miles away to Tampa because of advice from a policeman who was at my neighborhood shelter. There was only one domestic violence shelter with plenty of beds in the small town where I was raised, and I had to get away to be safe.

After I got here, I submitted applications to every safety net program I heard about. My application for long-term supportive housing has been granted because of my mental disorder. All of their waiting lists include me. I've been told that there will be a one- to six-month wait. I make multiple calls to every shelter each day in hopes of finding an opening.

I'm unable to work. I have excellent credit. I don't have any criminal history. It is irrelevant. I'm having a lot of trauma, and I'm finding it difficult to go through this process. A case manager can assist me. I've been informed that I'll get one AFTER my case is taken on by an agency with an opening.

I don't walk around thinking that I am owed anything by society. I just have no one, and I can't do this alone, so my only chance of surviving is through the generosity of strangers. I think there is a big hole in the middle of the safety net, and I have to face the fact that I might not make it. I'm fifty-eight years old. I have no idea how to survive on the streets. I'm afraid that the streets will take me and turn me into one of the crazy people pushing shopping carts while chatting to myself. Even though I'm fighting it, I'm not winning. It feels like I'm trapped in a terrible dream."

Pete

"I'm not here because I want to be. Nobody wants to sleep in a tent, on the ground, or on cement. Who would want to relieve themselves in public? Who'd like to smell something? Who wants to live in constant fear of being raped? Beaten up? Do rats scurry across your face while you're asleep?

Do you know what it's like to be dreaming and not sure of whether you are dreaming or waking up? It still amazes me that I'm really homeless. You keep thinking about what happened while trying to figure out what went wrong. That's how I felt my first week of homelessness a long time ago. I feel so alone now, as my family was the one who forced me to live on the streets after I lost my job during the recession. Back then, most of my friends were either still serving their deployments or had already left. I hadn't even moved out of town due to the recession two years before or even returned from a year in Iraq. Really, I had no one to help me. You realize really quick who your true friends are.

It's difficult, but I've gotten some survival skills. I rarely sleep through the entire night. In the beginning, I used to eat from dumpsters behind restaurants because I was always hungry. I wandered the streets, attempting to make out some sort of plan for my survival. I now follow a schedule, am aware of where to get food and water, and have made friends here on the street.

Consider this ... Even if you don't believe you could ever be in my shoes, consider what you would do if you were unexpectedly homeless."

Denzel

"Yo, imagine sleeping on a concrete slab instead of your comfy bed. Yeah, that's what it's like for some folks who are homeless. It's cold, lonely, and not exactly the definition of chill. Finding grub can be a struggle, too. No fridge full of snacks, just hustling for every bite. And showering? Forget fancy shampoos and hot water; it's more like baby wipes and the nearest public restroom. It's a tough life, man. People on the streets feel scared, unseen, and forgotten. But guess what? They're also strong and brave as hell. They face problems every single day and never give up hope. Peace."

Invisible in Plain Sight

My story of stories simply confirms that making the "invisible" homeless visible takes so little effort but makes such a big difference to the unfortunate souls living on the street. It's not about money. In fact, they never asked for anything during our time together. It's about seeing them, listening to them, and making them feel like real people with real stories. They deserve to be seen, valued, and heard. It's time for all of us to step up to make that happen "for good.

I cannot do all the good that the world needs.
But the world needs all the good that I can do.

Jana Stanfield

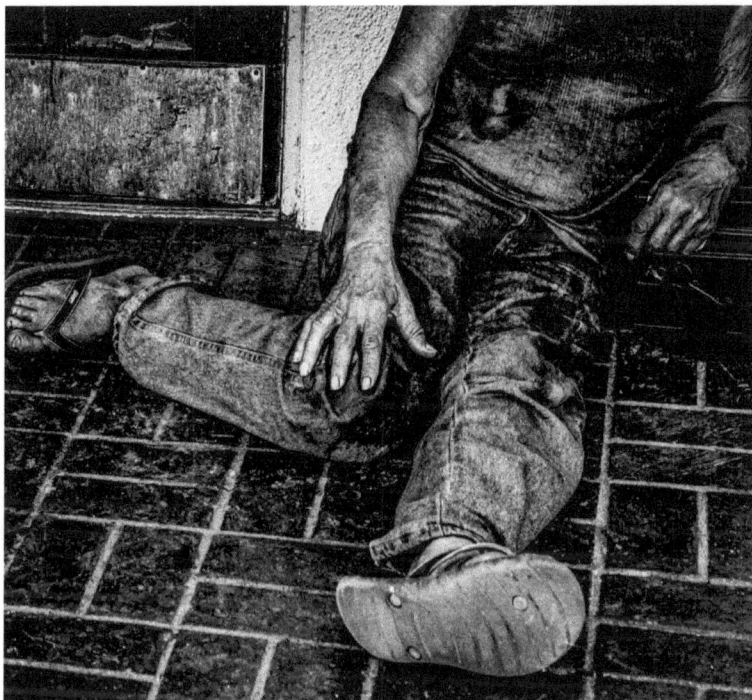

Dignity No Matter What: Collector Edition 2023
Renato Rampolla

Alone

(no backstory available)

Four Walls and a Door

By Amrita Valan
India

When I was 17, I came across this quote, which I have carried around in my heart since. *Whatever else they take from me, they can't take away my dignity.*

(Though they try.
And then I remind myself that they can't.)

I have never been unsheltered or homeless. Hence, it is probably the greatest fear of my life—something I transmit unconsciously to my children. Study hard, guys; you don't want to end up on the road now. This is a cautionary tale for those of us who live in India, the land of extreme *Haves* and *Have-nots*.

I know it sounds strange. I have had a privileged, sheltered upbringing in an upper-middle-class family in India.

India is a land of a vast populace and relentless migration of blue-collar workers in search of a better future in an exponential procession from rural to urban landscapes. Of refugees pouring in from the border to escape persecution, hoping not for any glittering Indian dream but simply to secure food to eat, clothes to wear, and a roof over their heads.

If lucky.

Daily, as I grew up, I saw homeless men and women still sleeping on the pavement or just getting up as I traipsed smartly to school in my crisply ironed, pristine white uniform, our maid in tow. Not to carry my satchel, as my mother made us carry our own school bags and bottles, but to protect me in those early years. In the eighties, horrendous tales circulated of kidnappers who lured kids away with promises of candy. The pathetic tale of *Billa Ranga*, two wealthy children abducted for ransom from school and then murdered in a botched operation, sent shivers through our spine.

Our parents purposely scared us, being themselves terrified. I was petrified when I overheard adults discussing the gruesome tale of a baby's abdomen stuffed with diamonds and sewn up to bypass customs and immigration to pretend it was merely asleep in "mother's" arms. What woman could do this to a baby?

So, we became completely indoctrinated.
"Never talk to strangers."

My big brother broke the taboo on our visit to cousins in Delhi. He not only spoke to a meek and harmless elderly beggar but gave him all the money he had, the princely sum of one rupee.

Oh, he was scolded so bad for it that I pitied him. What adults could evidently not see was seen by my brother and me—the hunger and helplessness in the unkempt old man's eyes.

His gratitude for a mere rupee.

But I was still wary, unlike my brother. Kidnapping was rampant in the eighties. Once, two men entered our building and approached my friend and me. They wanted to buy us sweets! My friend was five years old, a couple of years younger than me. She immediately agreed to go with a smile, but I pulled her away firmly.

But most of these old and infirm people were skin-and-bones rag dolls. Emaciated, starved-looking women with three, four, or even five kids were certainly not threatening. Nor were they an object of our pity, sadly. We had grown used to it, calloused by the hardness of our surroundings. We withdrew our eyes and went on our way, though as a child, it shook me to the core to see their living conditions. Mother often gave them alms, but there was a wariness.

**We had to remain careful because—
frankly, we were afraid.**

Often, there was nothing in common between us; many a time, the language was not our dialect (India is multilingual), and poverty did strange things to human hearts. Some hardened into criminals, capable of immense cruelty, even to babies. There is an underbelly of evil, a wickedness of human souls bludgeoned by poverty, hunger, and desperation, that to a child, appears unbelievable. We knew that children were often blinded or maimed intentionally by begging mafias to excite our compassion and earn them alms, which went to the extortionists. In return, they were fed and given "protection."

Once returning from school, I gave my guava to a street kid, who threw it away disgustedly, audaciously demanding money or cigarettes. Kids were addicted to *Beedis, a hand-rolled cigarette, because, often, the end of a hard day's begging fetched them, only a meagre meal or substance they could abuse.*

I have heard of kids sniffing glue and even downing cheap alcohol to alleviate the misery of their hell. That was how the racketeers kept them hooked.

A foreign returned friend had once scolded me, "You shouldn't give alms. It makes them lazy."

I felt intuitively that she was off the mark. The paradigm of honest day's labour and work ethics cannot apply to our vast country, which is not yet a first-world true welfare state. At least, it could not apply to children. And how could it apply to even adults when there weren't enough jobs to go around that paid well enough to keep body and soul together? We are a country known for cheap labour to the outside world. Cheap because many of us are forced to work for pennies since there is a substantial available labour force for the meagre quantity of jobs. It made no sense, and I could not exactly put it into words then.

I was only a first-year collegiate, but I remember saying, "At least when they try to earn it by rushing toward cars, at busy traffic intersections to clean windshields, or sell fruits, biscuits, or incense sticks, surely, they deserve our patronage." She had shooed off a boy attempting to wipe down the body of a car while I had reached for my purse automatically. My friend had been well indoctrinated in Western self-reliance but not the dignity of labour. I felt her scorn for my…well, "gullibility," and felt ashamed.

After I became a mother and cared for my own boys, it seemed to me our double standards were incredibly pathetic and absurd. So, I went into lanes to distribute books, toys, and old clothes, particularly to a beautiful young mother, a homeless woman with many small children, sprawling about on the road. The kids wandered around, dirty and bedraggled, with snot in their little noses. The mother periodically gave fierce love to her children, turn by turn, rather like a wounded tigress. I approached her timidly and handed her the two packages and a plastic bag I had brought.

She gave me a glazed, cynical look. Opening the bag, she smiled. As she brought out a few glossy picture books, her smile widened. She lifted her beautiful eyes, an incredulous mocking look in them, then threw back her head and laughed at me.

I could understand that the English books of *Tony Baloney* and *The Magic School Bus* were worthless to her. I wished I had brought her money and food. She took the clothes out and inspected them with amusement. I could not bear to watch her periodically giggle at my selection.

Thankfully, it was time to pick up my kindergartners from school. I rushed off.

No. I did not return. I guiltily looked at the mouth of the lane she bedded in but never entered.

We moved to an upscale special economic zone with luxurious high-rise apartments. Once more, daily, I witnessed the vagrant who lay apathetically on the pavement, a coughing emaciated guy with a horrendous beard.

In winter's cold, at 6 AM, I used to watch him shiver in his rag-tag threadbare blanket. At night, as I slept in my cozy Kashmiri quilt,

I thought and thought of him, my mind creating a rat's maze of terror where I kept imagining my own homelessness.

As an unprotected woman sleeping uncovered on the street, her babies being kidnapped casually by hoodlums (oh, the pity of affluent middle-class parents being terrified of the same), or being raped repeatedly and producing more helpless little ones.

Sometimes, I cried.

I imagined myself distributing blankets; what a joke when I was scared even to approach this man. I applauded the activists who collected old blankets and distributed them to the unsheltered in the winter. But I did not do anything. I sat in my beautiful home and tormented myself with my own insecurity, knowing that it takes but one wrong turn of fate to lose everything and stand where that incredibly beautiful girl was, denuded of dignity, out on the street, prey to nocturnal predatory men.

I have never been homeless, but I come close to tales of it happening to middle-class women, too, whose safety net of parents and family thinned out and disappeared as they grew old, infirm, or passed away. I have heard of husbands throwing out or abandoning wives and deserting children at such close quarters that it hit hard enough to hurt viscerally. And of elderly parents being pushed out into the streets, left at bus stands or pilgrimage spots, with promises of returning in a jiffy.

That jiffy never materialized. Becoming forever abandoned by wayside shrines, parks, and holy spots became their permanent fate. These once respectable but now deranged and destitute life givers became part of the homeless wandering mendicants.

Again, I have never really been "homeless," but I had come close to it when, in a moment of despair, I had run away. It had been a silly family spat. I wasn't an oppressed woman but a touchy new bride of three months. In a huff, I stormed out; while no one had asked me to leave, no one had stopped me either. Tears in my eyes, feeling incredibly helpless, I walked to the bus stop and took an old, familiar bus to my beloved university, my erstwhile hunting grounds. It was maybe four in the afternoon, and as the evening stretched interminably, I had time to cool off and observe the stray dogs circling me. I had been used to feeding them bits of my lunch sandwich, but that day, alas, I was empty-handed.

As it grew gradually darker, I shivered, realizing I was wearing flimsy indoor clothing, and my feet were shod in…my bedroom slippers! I shook my head silently as tears threatened to overcome my composure. That would have rung my death knell. Already, I could see an unsavory guy curiously ogling me with a look in his eyes that smacked of insolence. I wished I had sorted out my problems where they had begun, inside the walls of our safe apartment.

I was escorted back eventually. Sitting in a huff by myself on the stoop of my old college, watching the sunset in growing panic, I had done a lot of mental growing up. Life was not a drama fest, I had realized. Danger lurked in the guise of a hasty decision to run away from home, and now my night was out here, out in the open urban wilderness, without the comfort of family, a bed, or a closed door.

Then the headlights of my family car blazed in my face, and in a blind relief, I got up, tumbled into our car, and returned home in dead abject silence.

I was hurt, angry, and sullen.
I was also relieved and humbled.

How many, many women out there would count it a blessing to have this, what I had. Not a luxury flat, but the luxury of firmly closing a door to the outside world and taking shelter inside four hardy walls.

Amrita Valen ~ *Sincere Thanks to Dennis Pitocco for praising my writing and for the guidance and encouragement. Sincere thanks to my late mother and my eighty-plus courageous father, who has always provided me a home when I needed it.*

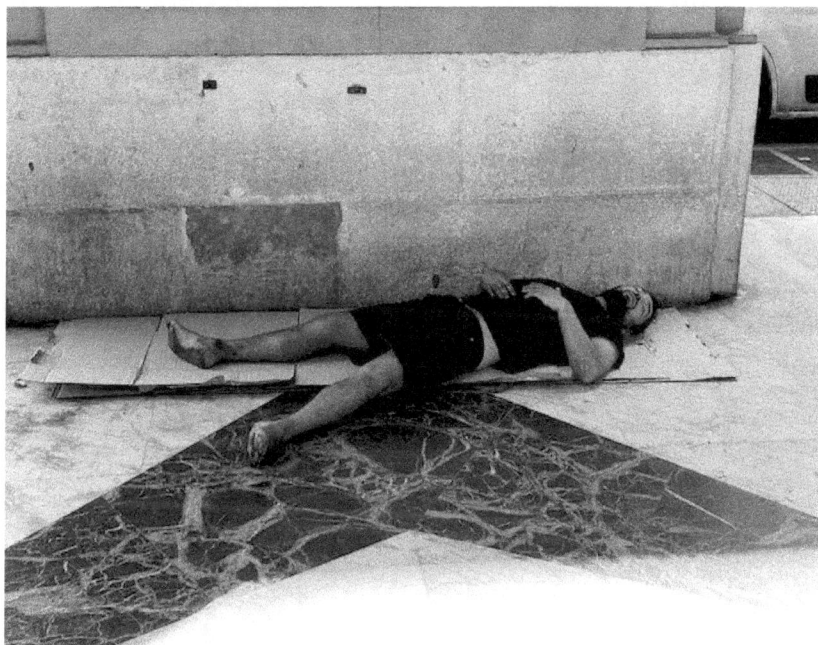

Florence, Italy
Dennis Pitocco, Photographer

A Wounded Journey From Survival to Self-Love and Self-Mastery

By Aneesa Theron
Cape Town, South Africa

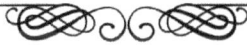

*W*hat does home mean to you?

Home, for the most part of my earthly existence, was about survival! Danger, destruction, emptiness, fear, loneliness, judgment, hostility, and negativity were deeply wounding and traumatizing to my precious heart. Escaping was always top of mind to find a place of acceptance and belonging! Searching for solace in other locations, friends, neighbors, and even the library, where I felt a semblance of normality.

Observing friends' parents and siblings who treated them with love, kindness, and respect gave me true examples of "home." I was grateful but more saddened and confused. I lived in six different houses before my 16th birthday.

I craved safety, peace, tranquility, and happiness!

I was dealt a harsh blow, exposed to perils with male predators under the influence of alcohol or drugs. I recall sharing my experience of molestation attempts in one of the homes where I lived. It was shrugged off, and I was mistreated as a liar fabricating stories. I vowed, "One day, my home would be everything I believed to be worthy of."

Is home a place or the people in our lives symbolize a good home? Though I had shelter, many times I felt homeless and would much rather have lived under a bridge or found safety on the streets. I do not wish my experiences upon anyone.

Almost daily, I was yelled at, fought negative energy, and was exposed to ugly and cynical chatter and frequent gossiping. I was frowned upon for being honest and authentic.

There were unfavorable expectations and entitlement to goodwill in the form of money, things, food, and whatever could be given free as a handout. As soon as I became independent, I was expected to make money and offer my earnings. I felt angry and appalled by this false belief and rebelled!

One day, my journal was missing. I recorded my deepest emotions, desires, dreams, inspirations, and fears. I felt hurt, angry, and betrayed. There was no remorse for their actions. I vividly recall tearing every single page into tiny pieces. Instead of nurturing, inspiring, and encouraging me, they were more interested in tarnishing my aspirations and disregarding my feelings. I chose not to journal after that experience until much later in my life when I felt safe to do so as an adult. I sometimes resist writing or journaling as this memory of betrayal and deception lingers.

Another embarrassing experience was when creditors knocked on our doors to collect overdue debts. The adults would hide and ask me to say they were not home. I loathed that I was included in their deceitful lies and that they never owned their responsibilities. They misled and fabricated stories just to avoid settling their debts. I pledged to myself that I would never be dishonest in this manner and would rather be responsible. Looking back, this particular experience shaped my relationship with money to the extent I feared not having sufficient and being in lack.

My maternal mom moved around a great deal, more than me. I often wondered why I could not live with her. She sometimes resided in a small room in someone's house. Or what we call a Wendy house, a wooden structure on someone's property. Though I never lived with her in these homes, I often missed her. When I was about 13, she moved into a small house with four of my siblings, and I pleaded with her to let me stay with her.

All that mattered was that I was finally home with my mom, where I believed I belonged. It was equally a relief being away from the hero/villain's home, where I was perpetually in a state of fight, flight, freeze, or fawn.

What I most enjoyed at my mom's was being with family, even if this was not always reciprocated or demonstrated with affection. I ached to be part of a wholesome home environment and not feel like an outsider.

Mom was excellent at cooking, and her eye for aesthetically pleasing decor; at times, I forgot we were living in a gang-infested neighborhood. Her strength and resilience to endure and overcome great adversity was another admirable trait.

Her struggles and trauma also showed up in the form of criticism, judgments, and aggressive tendencies while simultaneously presenting in victim mode. She also drank alcohol excessively and became a completely different person when heavily intoxicated. She once accused me of cheating with her boyfriend, my youngest sister's father.

**Her vicious outbursts whittled away
at my sense of belonging.**

While under the influence of alcohol, she displayed no interest in taking care of any of us. She lost interest in keeping our home clean and tidy, which she prided herself on. She always said, "Cleanliness is next to Godliness." Her binging cycles invited unsavory visitors into our home, placing all of us at significant risk of being surrounded by several strange drunk men and women, and in her heavily intoxicated state, she would leave our home for hours and sometimes days, leaving me with the sole responsibility of taking care of my siblings, cooking, and cleaning.

Our home was a 10-kilometer walk to school. The neighborhood experienced several abductions and murders. The police released a statement that there was a serial killer in our midst, preying on young children. There were no school buses, and I had no extra money to use public transportation. Due to the hero's house being much closer to my high school, I asked to move back as I could not bear the fear of the gangs and now a serial killer. It was for a short while only.

I moved to a place where I had much more freedom and my own room. The wife and I had a fair relationship and often communicated about various things. For the most part, I believed I would be content and settled until circumstances took a sudden turn for the worse.

Life became dreadful as the pressure mounted for me to contribute more financially. I was expected to pay more for rent, food, and utilities. At this point, I was doing casual work after school and on weekends as a cashier at a local supermarket. My chores increased significantly when I could not appease his wife with an adequate financial contribution. We never owned a washing machine, forcing me to hand wash everyone's clothing and bedding. I also washed windows, walls, and floors and ironed.

The turning point was during an evening when the wife was not home, and I was alone with a man who came in and out of the house. Let's call him the Jester, and I do not know why, but one day, he decided to introduce me to pornography. When he played a porn movie, I was immediately repulsed by his actions. Not only did he show me the movie, but he also asked me to demonstrate some of the acts, albeit the fact that we both kept our clothes on. I knew this was wrong; I felt an intense need to move from this house immediately, as my safety and dignity depended on it.

I have never shared this experience with anyone.

In my final year of high school, I stayed at a different neighbor's home with a couple and another male tenant with whom I shared a room. The woman of the house or landlady was quite firm with her rules, respected my freedom and privacy, and I never felt taken advantage of when doing chores. I was happy and at peace.

As I adjusted to my new surroundings, several incidents occurred, leaving me uncomfortable and fearful yet again. The woman's partner started to be suggestive, touching me inappropriately in passing or expressing flirtatious things to me. I never told his partner, fearing she would not believe me. Worse, I might be blamed for initiating it. I did not want to jeopardize having a place to stay, so I remained silent. The man I shared a room with became why I despised staying on. I never believed he would place me in an awkward, uncomfortable position.

Disturbing sounds woke me. I could see this man touching his private parts while he watched me sleep. I was an innocent teenager and felt nauseous, disgusted, and ashamed. I fled the home, though I questioned my role in all of it. Was it how I dressed, walked, or my friendly disposition?? What was the reason I attracted obscene, humiliating actions by these men?

I moved again, this time with a different neighbor on a familiar street. My favorite part of this home was that it was warm and inviting, but more importantly, I felt safe. I loved that the house was always clean and fresh, free from heavy cigarette smoke and drugs, as well as the heavy reek of alcohol. When there were celebratory days, the house was filled with family, friends, and activity. I experienced the most expensive seafood and meat dishes and dressed in my fanciest clothes.

It was amazing to witness a very different family way of life, which I was certainly not accustomed to.

After six months, I moved again; however, I always go back and visit. It keeps me connected to parts of my roots. The foundation may not have been solid, but it was a foundation.

This time, I moved in with a very close school classmate and her dad. This friend regularly visited the hero/villain's home, and we often met after school. I was familiar with their home and felt a sense of heaviness lifted from my shoulders. Still dealing with my despair and confusion about what had transpired at my previous residence, I was more alert and cautious around men. It was only my friend and her elderly dad staying together; her mom had passed on. Her dad was a business owner and spent most of his time at the office. This was somewhat comforting, having no adult men in our midst for whom I needed to be extra vigilant. Whilst it was fantastic having the place all to ourselves during the day, it was disconcerting in other ways.

The house was rarely cleaned, dirty clothes were piled up on the floors, dishes were stacked in the sink, and everything was unorderly. Neither my friend nor her dad desired a clean and tidy home. I was not sure if this was part of their grieving process after the death of their beloved mom and wife; hence, I felt obliged to cook and clean by myself. This became my way of payment as I was not expected to pay rent. Over time, my friend's character changed from a sweet, innocent young girl becoming rebellious towards her dad. She indulged in smoking, drinking, and eventually, boys visited, too. As teenagers, it was only natural for us to start showing interest in boys. Some of my friend's acquaintances were much older than us, while others were gang-related.

My friend also started working at a nightclub, and from there, we eventually drifted apart, and I sought new friendships. I wanted to steer clear of this environment. Even though I loved the space and freedom we had being by ourselves, I knew the dynamics at home invited trouble that would likely place my friend and me in harm's way. Yet I felt peer pressure to keep the peace and remained silent about my feelings. I focused on pleasing everyone, even though I no longer enjoyed or endorsed what was happening around me.

When a close friend suggested we move into our own place to start a new life independent of our parents, I jumped at the opportunity. I felt like a bird being freed from its cage. An escape from constant blame, shame, criticism, and judgment. Though in my final year of school, I was already earning money from my weekend job. Looking back, I can see that this girl in me was much stronger than I knew. She had the seed of self-mastery, fed and watered with time.

This town was even more rife with crime and drugs, plagued with many social ills. The social inequalities were apparent with many adults and kids walking the streets. Unemployment was high, and some parents could not send their children to school. Many begging vagrants accepted anything, offering some reprieve. Gangs surfaced on every street corner, and frequent fights broke out as they fought to claim their territory. I felt distinctively different from everyone else in this community—my light complexion and I dressed conservatively. I attracted lewd remarks and gestures from men. They would either whistle at me or move their lower body in a vulgar sexual way. I was uncomfortable and afraid, but I chose to disregard it.

Within a week, my school friend decided to move back home with her dad. This meant I now had a spacious room to myself. Although I was sad my friend decided to leave, I focused on my commitment to put myself first and leave behind a nasty, damaging life that consumed my former years. My newfound independence was liberating.

**I feared no one, felt no judgment,
and could live on my terms.**

Leaving home at 16, I inherited a few labels. The rumors were that "the apple doesn't fall far from the tree," implying I was destined to live a life of sin in the realm of prostitution. I escaped nasty bitterness and jealousy from an environment destined for failure and silenced the noise from my harsh critics. I was God-fearing and believed in the Almighty's divine plan for my life. I was young, but my optimism and faith soared me to greater heights. Though my time with my friend lasted only six months, it remains a positive memory and was a wonderful stepping stone on my journey.

From here, I was led to a new place of my own. I also started a new job in an upmarket mall. It was a blissful start to new beginnings in my search for better.

I am grateful in many ways today. Not only were my many experiences a training ground to become who I am today, but more saliently, they cultivated compassion, empathy, love, and kindness within me—a gift one can always celebrate amidst difficulties.

Fast-forward years later, I discovered home is within! A soul sanctuary is not something a single person can provide; neither has it access to destroy. When we build our place of refuge in people, it's an unfortunate recipe for disaster. Accepting all we are and loving ourselves unconditionally for our imperfections is the magic of a fulfilling life.

We choose to be a victim of our environment
or allow it to shape our life's direction.

Aneesa Theron

Aneesa Theron ~ *I am thankful for every person who contributed to me finding myself, be it through painful, shameful experiences, in addition to those who inspired and encouraged me to become a better version of that which I was born into.*

Interview with Marti MacGibbon

San Francisco Bay Area, California, USA

Vulnerable to the Bone

By Dr. Jo Anne White & Marti MacGibbon

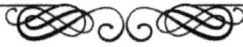

*T*hink about times you wake up in your house, and it is cold. Maybe there's a power blackout. You're maneuvering in the dark without lights or electricity, but you still have some control over your environment—candles, lanterns to light your way, and blankets to bundle yourself up. You have options. The heater went off, but you know it's only temporary: It's only a matter of time before the outage is resolved; the heat will resume, and you'll be warm once again.

Your mindset is that you don't have to endure this indefinitely, so it's easier to tolerate it. If a power outage occurs due to an extreme heat wave, and the air conditioner or the fans don't work, you're uncomfortably warm. Perhaps you decide to get in your car and drive with the AC on its highest setting to cool off until everything returns to normal. You may visit an air-conditioned shopping mall or grocery store on your drive to offset the unpleasant heat you're feeling.

However, when you're unhoused/unsheltered, you're exposed to the elements. It's an unrelenting fact of life. In summer, you're sweating or parched, or both. Winter ushers in the other extreme—bitingly cold temperatures, fierce winds that leave you shivering, feeling raw and bone-chilled. There's no relief in sight. You have nowhere to go to seek shelter, even temporarily, for some reprieve.

What if you wake up in bed at your home in the middle of the night and your stomach hurts? Maybe you didn't eat enough that day, and consider: "Should I get out of bed and fix something to eat, or just stay under the covers where it's warm and wait until morning?"

Think about times you get hungry or thirsty. You consider getting food delivered to your address. Instead, you decide to go food shopping. You get in your car, go to the store, buy what you need, leave, and drive home again. However, when you're unsheltered, those options are beyond your grasp. If you've been living rough, it shows. You're very conscious that you're unwelcome in the store unless you obviously look like you've got some money to spend.

Imagine yourself unsheltered: no address, no car. Out in the open and on foot indefinitely. You must keep moving, seeking a relatively safe place to sleep at night. If you find a bed in a shelter, you must get up at dawn and leave. Those are the rules. Maybe you look for work during the day, doing odd jobs. You're hungry a lot of the time. The state of being unsheltered is a state of extreme poverty. Maybe you had little to eat the day before and the days before that and counting. You're hungry enough to peer into trash cans or dumpsters in search of discarded food. For small amounts of cash, you may collect cans and bottles to recycle.

You are constantly living with the worry or fear that you could be physically attacked or even raped, perhaps by some young adults "having fun," by another unsheltered person, or anyone who sees you out there in the open, exposed, unprotected, and vulnerable.

When you lack shelter, you are also vulnerable to being trafficked, assaulted, and even murdered. You are defenseless. If attacked, you're not likely to report it. You hesitate to report a crime because you're committing a crime by being out on the streets: you're loitering, a vagrant. You're hoping to remain invisible to the police and to other people. A constant reminder gnaws at you that you're at the mercy of the elements and other people.

Being invisible isolates you; it increases your vulnerability and the risk of being attacked.

When you're "invisible," there are still eyes on you; there's no privacy. Where do you clean up, shower, or even go to the bathroom? How do you manage to hold on to personal belongings? What about your possessions? Where can you bury or hide your possessions or store them to have them when needed? With no safe recourse, you may have to carry them around with you. You're always in motion with nowhere to rest. The exposure you're enduring isn't only physical; it's also emotional and psychological. You never have a door you can close on the rest of the world, and you're doing things that you've never thought possible.

As other people drive by in their cars, you are keenly aware that they see you. Yet you can't really see them if they're in their car and you're just out in the open. There's never a level playing field. The vulnerability goes all the way to the bone. They may be thinking, as housed people often do, seeing unhoused people presumably acting strangely, that they're on drugs, drunk, mentally ill, or all three. Not knowing anything about the unsheltered person's past or present situation, they form harsh judgments.

Humans often have a way of deflecting and feeling safe and secure that this will never happen to them because they know better. Or since they've never actually met an unsheltered person, they assume this problem is something that only happens to a certain type of person. Thinking this way is reflexive; it relieves people of any thoughts of terror of being out in the street, unsafe and exposed.

Being unhoused can be someone's worst nightmare, and it could happen to anyone.

It could happen to you. What if you are a victim of domestic violence or lose your job with no immediate recourse to a salary or another job in the near future? Maybe you're dealing with a healthcare emergency or have experienced another sort of trauma or repeated life traumas. Perhaps you've just been released from jail with no recourse or backup. Or you're a youth who has been kicked out of the house, abandoned by family with nowhere to go. What if you're in an abusive situation that's so dangerous you're driven to escape to the streets? Everything breaks down: there are no resources and nowhere to turn for help and support.

How, when, and where does it all start? For Marti, the trauma began early on in her life. She was sexually abused at age fifteen by a school teacher. A victim of intimate partner violence, she fled, lived in her car, and was then sex-trafficked to Japan. It's not easy to put all that behind you. Often, people who've been sexually abused blame themselves, as Marti did. *Maybe I could have done something differently to avoid it, to get away.* That silent "if only" refrain runs deep, creating a body of self-depreciation that doesn't let up. Historically, the law and other people's judgments sided with the perpetrator. The "if only" catchphrase was blamed on the person who was the recipient of sexual abuse, which makes recovery and healing more difficult.

What if you became involved with someone you thought you knew? Someone you thought you loved only to find out that he was not that person. On the contrary, he garnered pleasure by being verbally, psychologically, and physically abusive. Where would you run to? How could you hide to get away from the incessant bodily attacks?

Marti ran to the street, to her car, to break free after being beaten nearly to death. Emergency staff at the hospital expressed surprise that she had survived the brutality. She drove nearly a hundred miles. Even that wasn't far enough to escape the man who was hell-bent on power, control, and vengeance. He stalked her. Whenever or wherever he found her, he assaulted her.

Being a woman outdoors, days and nights without friends or real connections, wasn't only daunting for Marti, it was outright dangerous. Every moment was a struggle to survive; finding calm, comfort, or self-assurance was challenging. Marti was always on the lookout for danger, not only from the abuser in pursuit but from the traffickers she had escaped, organized criminals for whom she'd be easy prey.

Living in one's car provides some shelter and a temporary hiding place. You could drive around so people didn't always see you in the same spot. Nor did they wonder what was up with you or decide to check you out. Unfortunately, when you're unhoused, the weather and external conditions can have devastating effects. They play a major role in your survival. When massive flooding occurred, Marti lost her car. There was temporary relief because places opened up to offer families food to help them through the environmental crisis. For a short while, Marti found access to clothing and food.

Yet even then, the trauma, loneliness, and isolation mounted. She was in a different category from the others. Marti was scared to reveal her circumstances lest someone betray her to the abusive boyfriend or the traffickers. After the disaster, families eventually received financial aid from FEMA to help with the damage to their homes and belongings. Some people were awarded trailers in which to reside. But that wasn't the case for Marti because she lacked a local address. It wasn't enough, even though she'd managed to hold on to her driver's license.

Once again, Marti was on the streets, on foot this time, with no relief from the elements or constant probing eyes. Clothes and other personals that were once stowed away in the car had been stolen by opportunistic thieves. Marti worked day labor to survive by chopping firewood, digging ditches, or working for a local landscaper pulling weeds and brush. She never panhandled because that would have increased her visibility and could prove fatal.

Despite carrying the trauma from her childhood, repeated sexual abuse, domestic violence, drug addiction, and being unsheltered, Marti endured. The heavy burden of it all could have destroyed her. But it didn't.

Marti is capable, intelligent, raised in an upper-middle-class family, and well-educated. When she was unsheltered, she had to strip away thoughts and fond memories of times she attended Shakespearian plays or films with her father. If pleasant memories of reading books or listening to classical music surfaced, she needed to push them away or bury them deep inside her. Marti couldn't allow herself to think about the "finer things" or her family. She reckoned that the pain, grief, and unfathomable loss would have been impossible to bear. Marti consciously and diligently resisted being pulled into the emotional abyss. Instead, she used her wits and focused on the present moment to survive.

But Marti didn't just survive. Eventually, opportunities presented themselves, and she thrived. Going from the depths of unsheltered life, she embarked on a new journey, receiving professional help and individual counseling. Marti obtained an education in chemical dependency studies and earned five professional certifications in the behavioral health field. She became a certified addiction counselor and case manager and taught classes part-time. Marti served as volunteer faculty at a women's jail for several years, teaching a life skills class.

Today, Marti is an internationally recognized humorous, inspirational speaker and bestselling author. Her nationally award-winning memoir, *Never Give in to Fear: Laughing All the Way Up from Rock Bottom, is a* gritty and humorous account of her journey through addiction. An empowered human trafficking survivor and advocate, Marti has spoken at the United Nations, the White House, the U.S. Department of State, the Department of Health and Human Services, and the Office for Victims of Crime.

You may say she was lucky, or perhaps she was different from those who were or are unsheltered, but that's not true. Consider what it takes to be unsheltered: the daily stripping away of the past, combatting and surviving with and against the elements, enduring hunger, sleeplessness, abandonment, and little or no support, respect, or true connection. Is that someone who is weak, lacking skill, or courage? No! That is someone with power, tenacity, strength, and resiliency, not just one person but the many people who've survived it all. They need to see themselves in a new light with dignity, and we need to see them differently, too.

Those tremendous abilities and skills can be channeled into work, helping others as Marti did and still does. She produced and performed comedy benefit shows for eight years. One hundred percent of the shows' profits went to nonprofits providing housing and other support for unsheltered people.

Having shelter is key, basic, and necessary. Where there is a lack of a solid and accessible safety net, people fall through the cracks and succumb to unsheltered living. Like many people who emerge from unsheltered existence, Marti wanted to be a part of the solution to help as many people as possible.

If you've been homeless for some time, reentry isn't easy. It's like starting all over, regardless of your age or status. The first step in rebuilding can seem monumental, especially if you're all the way down. You have to get an ID, which means you need a verifiable address for the authorities to mail the photo ID to you, as well as other documentation. An ID is also necessary if you want and need to hold down a job. That's where shelter and being housed come into play big time.

The human spirit has a tremendous reservoir of strength, resilience, and power, even if we don't believe in it for ourselves. Within us is this internal power we may not realize we have until we must. When pressing on in an impossible situation, despite incredible odds, that power rises. It's been demonstrated historically, throughout time, and even today amid the disruption of mass shootings, wars, poverty, discrimination, intolerance, and being unhoused.

Yet isn't it time for a global renewal or reset? Isn't it time to decide to harness this incredible reservoir that truly lives in all of us to make a difference and create a better world? There can be ways and means to help people even before they fall into this horrific predicament of being unsheltered.

For people who have been unsheltered, this core inner power can be utilized to motivate themselves. It's possible to draw strength and determination from remembering the adversities they have lived through and triumphed over.

It is wonderfully empowering to recognize that we can heal and recover from trauma. In the present moment, all of those dark experiences endured can be reframed as assets. All of us need to acknowledge that no matter what difficulties or traumatic experiences we've had, we are still standing and ready to move on.

Often, we hear about Post Traumatic Stress Disorder (PTSD), but we need to hear and learn more about Post Traumatic Growth (PTG). PTG has been defined as a positive psychological change experienced as a result of struggle with highly challenging life circumstances. The five domains of PTG are personal strength, new possibilities, relating to others, increased appreciation for life, and increased spiritual or existential meaning in one's life. People who've been unsheltered can emerge from the pain and suffering and regain a sense of hope, self-respect, self-satisfaction, and renewal. They can return to living life more on their terms.

We can all use PTG to shift our political, social, educational, and environmental systems and ourselves to create a better world. The question is how, and there are many forms and ways for implementation. The important response for us all is Now!

The Day My Life Shifted

By James Coleman
Myrtle Beach, South Carolina, USA

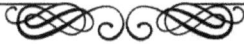

*W*hat do you see or do when you see an unsheltered (homeless) person? Do you turn your head and act like you didn't see them? Do you stare and thank God that it's not you? Do you think negatively towards them, like it's drugs, alcohol, or mental defect that brought them there?

The truth is that the reasons are as vast and different as the people who have found themselves without a place to call home.

Would it surprise you to know that there are doctors, lawyers, decorated military veterans, successful business people, moms, dads, grandparents, preachers, teachers, and children of all ages living unsheltered today?

Like many of you, I never gave it a thought. I chose ignorance and just turned my head and thought of drugs, alcohol, or mental defect. I often said to myself, "There, through the grace of God, go I," and just kept moving, acting like they didn't exist. Till one Saturday morning (in early fall) at church, when my whole life took a vastly different turn towards the unsheltered (homeless).

This is my story and how just one early morning act of kindness sparked a passion that I long to see fulfilled.

While I was attending my church's leadership program, my pastor pulled me aside and asked me if I would be interested in helping with the church's new homeless outreach program. As we talked, all I could see in my mind was being out at some homeless tent community passing out food and necessities or at a homeless shelter working a food line, and just thought to myself, "No."

Just as I started to feel guilty for even thinking about my response, my pastor dropped the vision bomb that would change my mind forever. He had a law enforcement background, and his son was a police officer in Columbus, Ohio. He explained the plan was not your typical homeless outreach. Our church would do something no one in our area had done before: bring the homeless to the church to serve them. Wait. What? What do you mean that you're bringing the homeless to church? Ok, I was intrigued! I had to check it out.

Saturday, October 6, 2000, at 6 AM
Still trying to wake up, I found myself pulling into the church. The pastor told me to come to the side of the church that had been remodeled over the last few months; it was now complete. As I entered the building, I noticed it looked like anything but a church. A large mural caught my eye with the scripture Mathew 25:40: "*And the King shall answer and say unto them, Verily I say unto you, Inasmuch as ye have done it unto one of the least of these my brethren, ye have done it unto me.*"

As I walked to the left of the mural, there was a small general store, and to the right of the mural was the entrance to a lounge area that led to a private shower and bath area. A set of wooden double doors in the center of the mural opened up to an elegant rustic dining hall centered from floor to ceiling with an early English stone fireplace. Ok, this was new!

I entered a large kitchen through the dining hall to find the pastor and a team he had put together. That's when he explained the vision.

"Today is about serving and nothing else. We have networked with several street evangelizing homeless organizations who will be bringing groups here so we can serve them. Once they arrive, the people will have the opportunity to enter the store, and they can select, at no charge, a new outfit and coat if needed, along with shopping for basic needs. Once they have finished, they can shower and enjoy the privacy of a private bathroom (10 in total).

Then, after they have finished shopping and cleaning up, they will be led to the dining hall entrance, where you will show them to a table and provide them with today's menu. You are to serve them and not evangelize to them. We are here to treat them as humans and give them a 5-star experience. After they have all been served, I want you to just talk with them and 'hear their story.'"

I couldn't believe what I was seeing and hearing. I started to cry as I realized that this was something no one had ever seen or done to my knowledge. This dining hall was something out of a magazine: 15 large round tables able to seat up to 15 people each, covered with a thick white cotton tablecloth. Centered on the table was a flower arrangement, and then there were 15 place settings consisting of crystal stemmed glasses, ceramic coffee cups, and the best in dining wares and heavy silverware. The menu consisted of several main dishes with side dishes, all breakfast or brunch style.

Our pastor led us in prayer, and from what I can remember, he asked each of us to have a servant's heart.

We began prepping and cooking what we could before the people started to arrive.

Saturday, October 6, 2000, at 10 AM
Buses pulled in, and the groups were arriving. Here we go!

We welcomed the first group and were assigned to small groups of four to six. I introduced myself and asked their names. Unfortunately, I don't remember theirs. Their nervousness and skepticism peered through their eyes. I respected that because I knew how nervous I was, and I was in an environment I was very familiar with. I reached out to shake their hands and introduce myself.

With a nervous laugh, I said, "I don't bite."

Some gave me a quick smile that faded as quickly as it appeared; others were expressionless, and some looked down at the ground.

One of the group asked, "What is the purpose of all of this?"

I responded, "It's something I believe you have never seen before, and I hope that by the time you leave, you will know people here care about you." My group all gave me a look of "Sure" with a visual tone of distrust.

"Let's go inside and get out of this cold, rainy weather." I showed them to the store, but before I could get my group inside, they all stopped and looked at the mural.

One person said, "That's beautiful, but do you believe it?"

Ouch, that was a tough question right off the bat. I responded, "Honestly, till today, I never thought about it. Honestly, I've been too busy just trying to care for my wife and son."

"At least you're honest," someone said. I thought to myself that was a good place to start.

As we entered the store, the group chimed in, "Is this for real?"

I responded, "Why, yes, it is. Take your time and get what you need."

After they finished, I took them to the lounge area and showed them to the private bathrooms so they could clean up.

My group looked at me, and one asked, "Who is paying for all of this and why?"

I responded, "It is our church's way of helping. It's a small gesture, just who we are."

After my group got cleaned up, we walked into the dining hall. The whole group stopped, and I immediately saw a lady (about 40ish) with a tear in her eye. "Are you ok?" I asked.

At that moment, I looked through their eyes. I recognized how overwhelming the environment was for those who lived on the streets every day with no place of their own, no idea where their next meal would come from, or even what it would be, and lived in a constant state of awareness or seeking protection. A tear welled up in my eyes. The gravity of our efforts was so much deeper than I expected.

As I sat my group at their table, one could see the bewilderment and awe in the faces of all the unsheltered as they looked around the room, stared at the place settings, and touched the crystal glasses and fine dining wares arranged in front of them. You could see life coming back into their eyes. I encouraged my group to take their time and review the menu.

I returned from the kitchen with a hot coffee pot and a pitcher of water and ice. As I walked around the table, filling their coffee cups and glasses with water, I watched them stare and slowly touch the cups and glasses as if bringing back memories.

After about 10 minutes, I began taking their orders, and almost simultaneously, they responded, "We can order what we want?"

"Of course," I replied.

One gentleman asked with a hint of shyness and shame, "May I have my eggs over easy?"

I fought a chuckle and replied, "You can have whatever you want on the menu and have it prepared however you desire." What had become so familiar and automatic for me was so foreign to them.

As I took their orders, our guests relaxed and let their guard down. As they began to open up, I could see smiles for the first time, and conversations started to erupt. The effects of this gesture of human kindness became more evident than I ever knew possible.

I went into the kitchen to help prepare the meals, and that's when the gravity of the situation hit me. My knees began to buckle, and I started to weep. Seeing these people feel normal and life come back into their eyes made me realize how much I had taken for granted, and it became more than I could bear.

We started to serve the meals and engage in conversations. After the food service, we mingled with our groups and listened to their stories.

It became quite clear as I listened that none of them wanted the life they were living. Economical situations were the commonality whereas drugs and alcohol were the rarity. The one story that stuck out the most was from an older man. This man (who wouldn't share his age) was a WWII veteran and was a lawyer for most of his life.

Then, as he described, a mishap in investments changed his whole world, and the life he spent creating fell apart within a moment as his investments crashed, leaving him broke. He lost everything. I asked about his family, and he advised he had none; they had all passed, and he had no children.

I realized very quickly that this group of "homeless" people was not so different than most of us. They once had dreams and aspirations and were not always unsheltered and alone. It was just a misstep in life that landed them where they were.

This experience placed a fire in me! As I travel for pleasure and work throughout the United States, I now have conversations with the unsheltered. I have learned to keep an open mind and take time to share a meal, a cup of coffee, or even a cigarette. I listen to their stories and see them for who they truly are—human beings.

Interview with Mercedes Wright
Don't Forget the Children

Rural Colorado, USA

By Peggy Willms

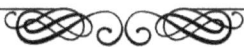

Why are you talking to me today?

I work for CASA (Court Appointed Special Advocates). We represent abused and neglected children within the court system ages 14-24 in rural Colorado. My clients are in the foster care system or have "aged out" of the system (those over 18), are at high risk for being homeless, or are currently homeless.

I want our youth to be healthy and happy. Age doesn't discriminate, especially when we are talking about our youth. This population is at a higher risk than adults when it comes to being homeless. They are in a crucial stage of development, do not have the necessary life skills to survive on the streets, are taken advantage of, or worse. And living in rural areas exacerbates the epidemic.

What is the most common reason this population becomes homeless?

Most become homeless due to an issue at home, whether it's domestic violence, physical, emotional, or substance abuse. Many feel safer on the street. Some fall into the foster care system, yet some run from foster care placement. The runaway youth tend to begin with couch surfing, whether with a family member or friend. If they do end up on the streets, they are quick to find or build a tight group of friends also living on the streets. Believe it or not, this can be a very compromising situation. There are cases with multiple people living under the same roof; some are under 18.

What are a few differences between homeless youth in rural areas versus those in major cities, such as San Diego or Seattle?

Just because a community is small, it does not equal small numbers or less of a problem. In cities, there are more agencies and amenities to tap into. Many small communities do not have soup kitchens or organizations offering blankets or other supplies. In our areas, there isn't enough funding to keep the shelters open year-round for adults nonetheless children.

Because of the lack of funds, shelters in our rural areas are only available from November to April. If the youth are not placed into foster care or aren't couch surfing, they are sleeping on the streets. Our temperatures drop as low as -10 Fahrenheit. We do our best to hand out sleeping bags and tents to keep them out of the elements. But it is never enough.

How does the foster care agency work for or against our unsheltered youth?

This is challenging. Number one, it is very difficult to place the teenage population. Most foster parents only want the little ones. The teenagers are "too difficult," which is one reason the youth run away. The Department of Human Services refers the youth to us at CASA, and we work diligently to find solutions. The runaway or homeless youth have unique issues compared to the adult population. Children are at the mercy of a guardian and cannot make their own decisions. Many children choose to remain a runaway versus being a foster child with the risk of having to go back to their original home.

This group is more clan-like and connect to those with a similar trauma or issue. Therefore, many try to stick together and avoid the foster care system altogether. This population is very emotionally sensitive, have abandonment and trust issues, and has a history of bouncing from home to home or relationship to relationship. Though they may find support with those with the same "issues," this can magnify the intensity of a problem.

You also work with ages 18-24. With low-income housing popping up across the US, how is this affecting this age group?
When a child turns 18, they "age" out of foster care. Low-income housing may be an excellent concept for those with low income or without a job, but there is still a gap for the children caught up in the unsheltered population. Many have not learned the skills to apply for or retain a job. Finding alternative housing remains a challenge. My boss started a tiny home project with one of our local construction companies and a team of other professionals. Habitat for Humanity allowed us to move it onto their property to work on it.

Our goal is not only to provide shelter but also to utilize our unique mentorship program. Many have not been exposed to environments with proper education, healthy habits, or a positive support system, so we put together a team of experts to help. The bottom line is that low-income housing still requires "income."

What is your experience in teaching them life skills?
They lack confidence and self-worth. They are raw. Not only are many exposed to physical and mental abuse, but they have also witnessed or participated in illegal behavior. Mental health or substance issues run rampant because some of this population is born into or grew up in an unhealthy environment—learned behavior. Finding care or solutions for this population differs from finding solutions for adults.

We have found that many youths have not seen professionals and have gone undiagnosed. There are a few reasons: 1) their parents or guardians have taught them that health care providers are evil; the parents do not want the heat to come back on them, and 2) they are afraid to be tossed into the foster care system. We often start from scratch, teaching them hygiene, cooking, and how to fill out applications. This is done in our weekly meetings.

Do many leave the home with a parent and begin living homeless?

Some do. In most cases, it is to escape domestic abuse. A homeless teen was living in a car with his mom. She is a heavy substance-abuse user, and unfortunately, he is also using. We placed him in one of the houses we built, but he is still struggling. I see him three times a week, but because he is on drugs, he remains on the streets.

We know we can't expect someone to quit immediately, but they still need a roof over their head. This is an excellent example of a catch-22. How can you help someone who doesn't want help? Though families do end up homeless together, many of the children age out of the foster care system, and most remain homeless.

How do youth find the system's services if adults have difficulty themselves?

This is a huge problem. Many outreach programs are outstanding. But we realized "we had to go find them." I'm going to the schools, pastors, and community. We need more public events explaining what is available. We need to take to the streets. For example, since 2007, November has been dedicated as National Homeless Youth Runaway Prevention Month (NRPM), yet many haven't even heard of it.

During this month, some schools collect and offer supply kits such as hygiene items, canned goods, and blankets. They wear purple on Fridays. But again, what if the child isn't going to school and lives in a rural area? They don't even know how to access these "perks" in November? Large communities such as Denver advertise this program, but rural areas often do not have the funds to advertise; therefore, many of our youth never hear what's available.

We must find the underserved children. Listen to them. Building a rapport and gaining trust is our immediate goal. Even if we can only provide them one meal that day, we must be OK with that. We won't fix the whole problem and save the world in a day. It is about due diligence and consistency, which sometimes means providing things that buck up against what society says is the solution. Some cases are unique, and cookie-cutter approaches don't work. Giving someone a pair of gloves doesn't mean you are condoning their situation. It means you want them to be warm!

You have shared that rural areas differ regarding lack of local, state, and national publicity, access to funding, experts, and more.

Building a rapport with them is the most successful approach. This population struggles with critical thinking and has less follow-through. Many revolt and see the help as control, just as many teens do. Most have a 13- to 14-year-old mentality, and some as low as five. We also reverse-teach, trying to unravel what they have already learned from their parents and guide them to healthy choices and life skills.

They are also at risk for multiple partners, which increases the odds of transmitted sexual diseases and multiple pregnancies; they are not seeking medical care and are not skilled enough to take care of themselves, never mind a baby.

What does crime on the street look like for the homeless youth?

There is a lot of behind-the-scenes crime. There are many reasons someone commits a crime, and I am not stating crime is excusable, but many youths shoplift for necessities like socks, warm clothes, or food. However, some homeless adults will "pimp out" the youth to steal items or to perform sexual favors creating income for the adult.

Many kids say the older homeless population hurts them and takes advantage of them, knowing they can use the system against them. "If you don't do this. I will turn you in." Unfortunately, the flip side is that some youth will learn this behavior from their elders and begin mimicking it as they age.

We know that finding a purpose in our lives, a reason to get up and make a difference, is one of our basic human needs. Are you addressing this area with your youth?

This age group is extremely creative. They write poetry, music, paint, and more, but again, they must be praised for doing so and given an environment or tools to improve their talents and gifts.

We are trying to offer them nights such as Movement Monday and Open Discussion on Wednesdays to discuss various topics such as LGBTQ+. We also have Game Night on Fridays. Supporting and giving them a safe place does wonders for their relationship building, reducing stress levels and building confidence.

What is your experience with collaborative efforts between agencies in your area?

I want to commend all the sources that are working together. Teachers are important because they are exposed to these kids for several hours daily. They know, more than we do, who does and doesn't have a home or a safe home. Who does and doesn't eat or bathe? We need to reach out to each other more and capitalize on the strengths of each agency.

Some feel homelessness is a lost cause. What keeps you going to work in this profession?

Knowing I can make a difference. We all can. In my personal case, I understand where they are coming from because of my life experiences, and I have always wanted to help people. This population is different and underserved. That is what keeps me going. It is my privilege to work with and watch these kids grow.

Many have been forced into their situation, and I am blessed to be a part of not only changing their current lives but changing the future they would have had. They might be troublemakers because they have had to defend and fend for themselves. Most of them are good human beings who haven't had a chance and just need an opportunity. Most teens overlook the privilege, luxury, and benefit of having someone who loves them, provides for them, and keeps them safe.

If you had an audience before you who are not homeless, what would be the call to action you would give them?

Educating and helping unsheltered youth, at least in our rural area, is about building rapport and trust. Once they feel safe, it spreads by word of mouth to their friends. What they learn from us, they repeat.

Do you know the stats in your community, what services are offered, and where are the gaps? Find out! Every community is different. There isn't one approach that works across the board. Increase your knowledge about homelessness in general: why are youth becoming homeless, what strategies are working, and what ones are not? What can you provide to decrease the number of these underserved youth?

Speak to your law enforcement agency or schools and ask how you can help. Volunteer your services, teach writing, painting, or other creative classes. This population uses creativity to express themselves, and many are very talented. Write to your local, state, and national representatives. Homeless youth require similar services as adults, such as doctors, counseling, safe houses, food banks, etc., but they require different approaches when you are advertising your services. They are confused, scared, and do not know how to cope.

We need more publicity by news, radio, print, and social media. If you are a teacher, look for the signs! Many homeless youth are picked on or outcasts, some smell because they haven't bathed, or eat quickly because they are starving. Think outside the box. Hand out water, granola bars, blankets, sleeping bags, tents, gloves, hats, etc. HAND THESE THINGS OUT. They will take them even if they cannot use them themselves, and they will offer these items to those who can.

You are not "adding" to their homelessness by putting food in a belly or preventing hypothermia. Also, teach our youth about the unfortunate youth. Our judgmental youth of today will become judgmental adults, and homeless youth are likely to become homeless adults.

Final thoughts?
We cannot turn the other way with this issue. We are not going to improve the adult homeless population if we do not start looking at the youth who will eventually fill their shoes. Every demographic is affected by the homeless, whether you are actually homeless yourself or not. It affects every ethnicity, location, health condition, and economic status. It can happen to anyone. Learn More – Do More.

We are all struggling to make ends meet. Imagine you are 14 and must leave home with only the clothes on your back. Where will you sleep tonight? Where would you find safety? What dumpster would you pull out a half-eaten Big Mac from? Tonight, most teens are studying for a test or getting into trouble for not picking up their room. Tonight will be very different for the homeless youth population.

Turning our heads on the adult homeless population is one thing. Turning our heads on our homeless children is despicable!

Off the Street on Our Feet

By Mathew Broster
Byron Bay, NSW, Australia

Money in the right hands can change the world.
Money given to the right hands can heal the world.
Money with the right plans can redeem the world.
There has never been a better time to
change, heal, and redeem our world.

Mathew JC Broster

*A*fter recently being homeless and fresh from an intense few weeks in an acute mental health facility in early November of 2022, there I was, out in the real world.

Whether seeking happiness and buying a one-way ticket from London to Asia ten years ago or turning to drugs, psychedelics, binge eating, or alcohol, I allowed escapism and addiction to rule my life. Seemingly, even when I "have it all," I have a problem. Mainly via secret binges, and while being too afraid to admit my lack of control or how I was constantly filling a void, my awareness of these truths only seemed to make things harder.

I was one of the lucky ones, though. When I was sectioned in that acute mental health facility, I had a visit from a homeless organization that tried to shelter people like me. Within a week of being discharged, and after some more tent time (living in a tent), I moved into an emergency-sheltered accommodation in Byron Bay, NSW, Australia.

By early March of 2023, my depression was as severe as ever, my anxiety left me frozen in all social situations, and my hidden and psychosis-based problems were extreme. After several weeks, in the midst of an intense mental health assessment, the head psychologist, who had never spoken to me, abruptly halted my mental health assessment. My mental health concerns were deemed "too complex," and my chances of being further diagnosed were stripped away. Even after multiple requests, he wouldn't speak with me, which significantly hurt me. I felt deeply abandoned, pushed aside, and not taken seriously.

My chances of being officially diagnosed and receiving the proper care I needed cruelly vanished.

Along with my diagnosis of Borderline Personality Disorder, Complex PTSD, Bipolar Disorder, and Generalized Anxiety Disorder, I was about to be taken seriously and be properly diagnosed with ADHD and Delusional Disorder. Since being diagnosed with Bipolar Disorder in 2016, I have been on and off antipsychotics. Except for medication, I had never been thoroughly evaluated. His flippant decision to terminate my testing increased my suicidal ideation dramatically.

Did anyone care? Did the system fail? Or both?

I was just another mental health tag to dismiss. Another number of many swept aside. Another broken human who loses their power while trying to heal. And all because of a title assigned to them. Things need to change. Enough is enough.

Honestly, it is a miracle I haven't ended my life. The intense mental health assessment, which included my family, was hard enough just to be severed at the last minute. I'm not surprised that suicide is the most prolific pandemic in our world. I am determined, though it feels like a living hell daily, that I can be a voice for many who go unheard, who are left to fight alone, or who have ended their lives due to hopelessness.

In early March of 2023, I lay in bed, depressed and contemplating how to best end my life. I forced myself to go for a run. On this run, and similarly to the psychosis, I went through back in 2019, when I publicly expressed how I thought I was Jesus and even published books about it, I was hit with an unseen force. Though, on this occasion, it was not as extreme as receiving messages that I was the "second coming."

This unseen energy felt divine and angelic yet not nearly as far-fetched as it had been on previous occasions. The surrounding trees in the beautiful forest were talking to me. If not them, maybe angels. However, these visions were extremely confronting and charged with emotion, logic, and realism. Yes, they would most certainly seem farfetched to the average Joe, but somehow, I knew they could come true. The only thing that would prevent these visions from coming true would be me.

Despite my ridiculous amount of social anxiety and feeling incredibly awkward in social situations (hence being single, being petrified of intimacy, and not having any real close friends), I knew I could not disregard this vision. In a nutshell, this seemingly angelic force took over my body, mind, and spirit, and with tears of fear, courage, proudness, and apprehension all running down my face, the vision was then given. The vision unfolded in a whirlwind of images, feelings, knowledge, and voices.

The Vision

The vision was to get acquainted with homeless people from a local homeless hub and encourage them to start running with me three times a week. We would train for an upcoming Gold Coast marathon event just a few months away. We would have a running coach on each run, a running plan would be created, and our training would intensify—running barefoot with dogs on the beach, increasing to hill runs while whales breach, and even longer runs in the rain. I saw and felt it all. I felt the breakthroughs. I felt proud of my achievements. I felt successful.

During this whirlwind of divine intensity, I could feel the innocence of our runners, those involved, and even of me. Despite the ongoing battle of "No, I can't do this" and "Yes, I can do this," I could see the hurdles jumped, the spirits touched, and the hearts warmed. I envisioned the depths of their personal achievements, and it brought me to tears. It was as if many of them were so deeply scarred that they had completely lost their identity, me included. For the first time in our lives, we would finally get at least a glimpse of our true selves. We would finally see our radiant beauty hidden behind the trauma, beyond the lies, beneath the pain, beyond the abandonment, and above the worthlessness.

What I felt, saw, and knew was intensely beautiful, unconditional, compassionate, and giving, just like a harmless child—lovable purity, the sweetness of innocence. Yet, this hidden beauty was so petrified of the world and society; all things were a threat.

Even though it's very difficult to put into words, I felt the true nature of humanity, the true humanity of those I could see going from the streets to the finishing line. I felt their authentic essence, internal spark, and undeniable divinity. In reality, I didn't know any of the souls I was feeling, nor could I see their faces. I just knew that what I saw in them, I also saw in myself.

I realized at that moment that shards of glass surrounded our hearts. These shards of glass made it impossible for us to truly trust, truly love, truly accept, and truly love ourselves. Beneath the shards of glass preventing our true hearts from a beautiful start was the most fragile child. Infused with childlike enthusiasm, wholesome fun, endearing excitement, and the wildest of innocent love, I could feel it all.

Unfortunately, the fractured brokenness that had become a crumbled soul had many layers. Humanity may see this suppressed brokenness as victimhood, addiction, laziness, anger, and even abuse, crime, and/or bad behaviors. However, what I could see deep down was enough to bring me to my knees in tears. My innocent tears of many emotions streamed down my face, and I felt something so incredibly rare. My heart opened. As I had stopped running amidst this divine intervention in such a beautiful forest, I hoped no one else would come through at that moment. I was experiencing something I couldn't explain.

Along with the purity of what I believe is in all of us, the unconditional beauty I saw in the souls who crossed my path opened my heart, giving me faith in humanity. I could no longer question or deny what I felt, especially for those left feeling abandoned, rejected, unsheltered, and consumed by surviving and not thriving. This vision intensified more than I could have imagined.

I then saw the trophy. I saw a local celebrity (Chris Hemsworth – Thor). I saw team singlets and jerseys. I saw us in proper running shoes. I saw us raising money for the homeless hub and a team awards presentation. I saw myself as a community role model and receiving recognition. I saw the media supporting us. I even saw us on TV, in local and national newspapers, in magazines, and in the news. As the visions flashed one by one, so did the emotions. The feelings of this personal and humanitarian achievement were second to none. Both are magical yet somehow realistic. I saw, felt, and was immensely emotional by the proudness of the community. Hearts were touched, and even those who once walked past the homeless now had a connection with them.

It was as if I was watching the best clips of an uplifting movie that had touched the hearts of the homeless runners, the community, the nation, and even the world. As part of a secondary vision I write about in my upcoming book *From a Mental Health Ward to a Nomination Award*, I also felt that a movie would be made of our story one day. Being that I feel that mental health sufferers are the greatest actors ever known, I may even have a chance to be involved.

It was astounding. I saw people from awful backgrounds come off the street and be kitted up as a team of legends. It was incredibly emotional and beautiful seeing these individuals feel proud of their achievements and being recognized in the newspapers, magazines, social media, radio, and TV. The community was joyous and felt a part of their journey.

This vision extended beyond homeless people breaking stigmas, judgments, and stereotypes as they empowered themselves by running in a marathon event and for their homeless hub. It was a chance for all walks of life to see the true humanity in all people regardless of their class, status, lack of a home, or separation from mainstream society. It was a chance for so many of us to experience togetherness, epic comeback stories, and unity like no other. It was a chance to see those left on the street, recovering addicts, and many who have experienced homelessness or those at risk of actively getting up and making something of themselves, me included.

The Reality

The vision came true—our first official training run was on April 12, 2023, and the big day of the Gold Coast Half Marathon was July 1, 2023. Reality was more significant, incredible, and astounding than that of the mind-blowing vision I received while running in early March of 2023. Running between rough sleepers and Olympic athletes along the beach of Byron Bay while whales breached and Swedish TV filmed us was a reality. It happened.

Our 11-week running program was created for us by the Australian under 23's head coach, who accompanied us throughout the journey. I hosted the official "Off The Street On Our Feet" awards presentation, showcased to an intimate audience. Our audience included local community members, business owners, an Olympic medalist, local churches, sponsors, board members, our team, and more. The entire team of Byron Bay Runners coached us from start to finish and became lifelong friends. They were also presented with a signed and framed singlet. One of our homeless runners had found an old 1996 horse racing trophy. An amazing lady in a local trophy shop transformed it, and it has become our very own "Off The Street On Our Feet" trophy.

Most of all, a combined team of 22 participated in the 2023 Gold Coast Half Marathon. This included our core team of twelve, two staff from the homeless hub (Fletcher Street Cottage), and ten runners from Byron Bay Runners Club. Just as the initial vision had shown me, we were on the TV (ABC News). We were also on the radio (ABC News Radio, Bay FM, BBC Radio, and Faith FM), and we will be featured on TV twice in 2024, as well as in *Rolling Stone* magazine and BBC radio.

As for the individual stories that came from our core team of runners on that memorable day, the personal breakthroughs were magical. The comebacks, the rewritten stories, and the self-discoveries, all in the face of adversity, were phenomenal: After no sleep whatsoever, we had one homeless guy who started the race in his dressing gown. While being high on psychedelics, and despite no training whatsoever, he achieved the finishing time that I had trained 11 weeks to get.

To me, that shows something inside of him that is extremely powerful. Seeing him walking around Byron Bay proudly wearing his finisher's T-shirt and with his medal around his neck was heartwarming. When he saw me, he thanked me, hugged me, and repeatedly said how special I was and how proud he was.

There were such monumental achievements from many who were unsheltered. A disabled guy who was born with backward feet finished the entire 21km. A woman went from paralyzed to finishing the race. A recovering addict ran the event in the shoes his Dad left him when he died from cancer. And a tent-living person finished the race in an astounding 90 minutes. How about the guy who almost had to run handcuffed to his parole officer? Yep, that happened, too. Or the unstoppable legend recovering from a heroin addiction, and after having two strokes and dying in the hospital, he defied death twice, came back to life, and finished the race.

There were many moments similar to this where I had to hold back the tears. My heart softened as I learned their personal stories, no matter how hurt I felt. None of us will ever forget what we overcame that day, including angelic moments and breakthroughs.

The Outcome

I had another vision in late September of 2023, after another four running events, including a mountain peak run, full marathons, and even a 36-km run. This time, it was during a dream as I slept. From that dream, I immediately flew to the UK.

My situation was the same as in February 2023, but now it is a year later. Returning to my hometown was a big deal because I openly and very publicly thought I was Jesus back in 2019-2022. As déjà vu would have it, during this most intense psychological battle, I wish it was just a bad nightmare. But here I am.

Just like in February/March of 2023, spending days frozen in bed, too afraid to live, too lethargic to do anything, and absolutely terrified of being around people, here I am in a similar situation but a year later. Can I do all this again and perhaps still disregard my mental health? Is it a sign that I have to go it alone and that I never seem to get any help because I can do this? Is it part of my own redemption to follow this same unseen path towards a farfetched vision too large even to mention?

This story is just a partial glimpse of my surreal journey, especially since my massive awakening/psychosis in December 2019. My memoir, *From a Mental Health Ward to a Nomination Award*, will be published in the coming months. What about Chris Hemsworth? What happened next? What about the secondary vision? Yep, there was even more to the initial vision, which I will explain in my book.

I still can't logically explain my journey apart from it being miraculous and that it is still ongoing. My mission is to share my experiences and those of others as we strive to come off the street and on our feet.

Mathew Broster ~ *Without the Byron Bay Runners, the community, the media, local donations, and even Chris Hemsworth (Thor) approaching me, this would have never reached the success it did.*

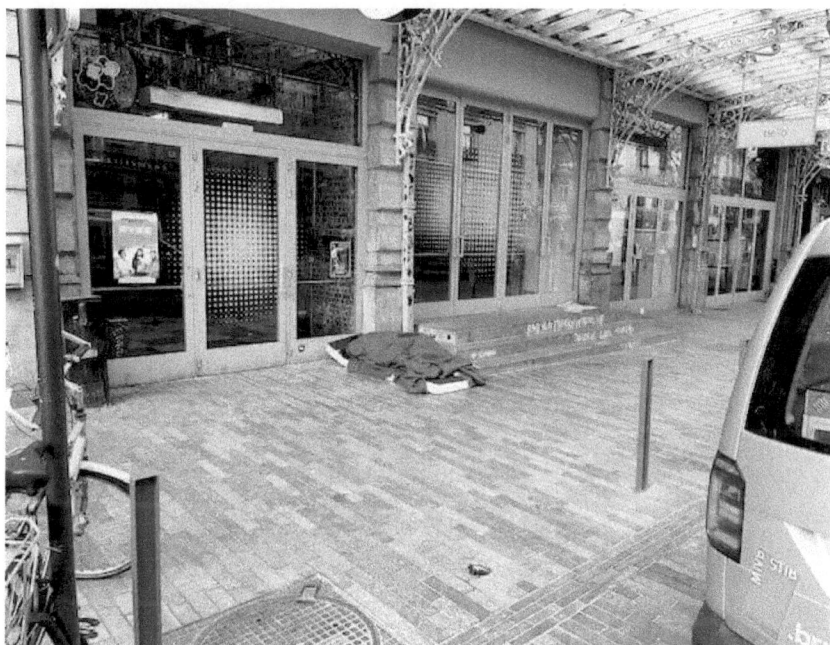

Brussels, Belgium
Dennis Pitocco, Photographer

The Final Chapter

By Julie Winkle Giulioni and Paul Wright
(In memory of Don, Los Angeles, California, USA)

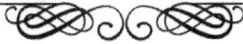

*W*hen my brother Don and I were growing up together, I became his voice. Although learning to speak came a little later than usual for Don, that didn't stop him from speaking a kind of gibberish that somehow I managed to comprehend. That was how my brother and I became able to communicate, granting me the privilege of becoming his interpreter to the world until the language he heard around him could become his language, too. Being another person's voice may seem like having a passport to their mind. Yet that gift never helped me answer the endless questions, and the mystery persists four years after Don's death – especially questions about his homelessness.

Understanding homelessness is challenging in and of itself, and the more I reflect on his life and my memories of him, the more the complexity and nuance persist. Telling the story may not uncover answers. But it definitely helps to see the questions more clearly.

I wish I could say that there was something special about our life at home with our parents, but there wasn't. Don and I shared a stereotypical upbringing in Southern California. Our mother was a highly-engaged PTA mom who took us to school and was there when we returned home each day, while our father held two jobs as a printer to provide for us. Although we had a comfortable life, we were less financially secure than those around us. For our family, there was always a subtle pressure to "keep up."

We jokingly referred to our community as "Mayberry." A town where people looked out for each other and knew everyone's children. If I ever did anything amiss on my way back from school, my parents likely knew by the time I arrived home. Did we have our dysfunctions? Of course. But I couldn't imagine a more supportive and stable foundation to launch the lives of two children.

Like most of their peers, our parents wanted to provide more for us than they had. This was the case with education – they were committed to ensuring my brother and I had a fine education. This was important because Don was brilliant – likely with a genius-level IQ scale. He was also naturally athletic and excelled in any sport he tried. He even played ice hockey well into middle age – when he could.

I was a year and nine months older. It's not a significant age difference, but nonetheless, I found myself taking on a protective role in his life. This was how I came to serve as his "interpreter," trying to translate his babble into something understandable for our parents and others. As our paths diverged later in Don's life, I kept a keen eye on him, although it became a more complicated role to fulfill.

Shortly after college, my brother ended up on the streets for the first time. I suspect drugs were involved. But Don always seemed driven by aspirations that simply didn't match his ability to make them real. It may have been this frustrated desire to live beyond his means that led him to make poor choices along the way, which caused him to just disappear for about six months, leaving everyone with no idea of what was happening to him.

While he was radio silent, I'm also guessing he experienced a lot of fear for his safety, as well as shame and embarrassment. Pre-cell phone era, we were left anxiously waiting until he resurfaced. Not knowing if he was dead or alive was excruciating for our parents.

When he did return, he never shared
his personal life with us.

Occasionally, with hard-to-fathom ways of telegraphing his presence, he would suddenly surface like one Christmas Eve when a poinsettia plant and card appeared on our front porch, letting us know he was alright. Reflecting on that memory, I interpret Don's sweet gesture as his way of letting us know that he was "okay." But it also highlighted an ongoing dissonance. At his core, he remained himself, and yet, he was living an unimaginable life and facing dangers we couldn't even conceive.

In hindsight, this "first disappearance" can be read as a foreshadowing of what was to come. As abnormal as it seemed, my brother was adept at returning to what outside observers might construe as normal behavior (like delivering a holiday plant.) In fact, despite all the dysfunction clearly at work in the background, later in life, we all (including Don) managed to maintain oddly "normal" interactions in keeping with the social norms of everyday regular reality. But always with a twist.

Finally, he reached out, knowing he needed help to lift himself from the depths he'd sunk to. He hit bottom at the Circus Circus Casino, where he subsided on popcorn and coffee for some time. (Years after his time on the streets of Las Vegas, he had an aversion to eating popcorn.)

My parents sent him a bus ticket on the condition that, once he was home, he would proceed directly to a nonprofit program called Union Station Homeless Services. Union Station's core emphasis at the time was drug rehab, but it now provides housing and the support to hang on to it. It also helps residents achieve stability as they re-engage with their community. It certainly seemed to work for Don, helping him return to something like "normal."

At the time, Don seemed to be an inspiring story of recovery, a narrative that showed him regaining his life, returning to his family, and returning to something that seemed relatively normal. Even in writing this and using the word "normal," I can hear the judgmental weight the word implies. To be clear, I use it to depict an existence involving relationships, having a job, paying, bills, and taking a shower – activities we're taught to reflect a certain routine quality about our lives. And so, at least by outside appearances, that was my brother's life for the next 30 years.

Until he, once again, found himself living on the streets. (What I understand now is that homelessness is not a simple binary condition – not either black or white, on or off, in or out. There is a lot of gray. The transition from being housed to unhoused is as difficult to discern as it is to single out one day and say, "That's the day it happened." Yet, looking back, I believe that for the final six or seven years of Don's life, there was never a consistent roof over his head.)

During those 30 or so "normal" intervening years, much of Don's life revolved around work. Like our dad, he had a remarkable work ethic, loving to jump into a challenge, share his talents, and make a difference. He was fearless in the face of hard work and was elevated to two management positions with significant responsibility. And just as in most normal work environments, Don enjoyed some close friendships.

He engaged with our family and my children, who adored their uncle thanks to his humor and zaniness. This was especially helpful because his willingness to watch over the kids allowed me to return to school and finish my degree. I couldn't have done that without his support, and I will forever be grateful to him.

Over the years, his housing grew increasingly unstable. My husband and I found ways to help him, including allowing him to stay in a small house just behind our home. Ultimately, we helped Don move into his own townhouse. But alas, it didn't last, and my brother moved into that grey zone between being housed and not. Interestingly, his dog seemed to be a stabilizing force during that time. Don was more concerned about Hank's comfort and safety than his own. But once Hank died, so did Don's commitment to housing.

Having gone through the experience of homelessness once much earlier in his life, perhaps Don could see the choices before him, in a sense. Becoming invisible was one of them. With homelessness came invisibility. But gratefully, with more regular family contact this time around.

I remember Don describing how he found a place to pitch his tent, where he could keep his possessions safe. He seemed proud of coming across a nook in the hills that other homeless people (and officials trying to eradicate homelessness) wouldn't find. He had a way of speaking cryptically – likely to spare me the details that would only worry me. Yet, he'd often invoke his wicked sense of humor as well, weaving tall tales that made us laugh until we cried.

I vividly remember a dinner out where he had us rolling on the floor laughing as he regaled us with a story about "wrestling" a raccoon that had gotten inside his tent one night. We'll never know if it was true. But it was just like him to wrap up whatever was happening in a sense of normalcy, perhaps to keep us comfortable, hoping that it made it easier to overlook that he was unhoused.

And, of course, I never saw him in that "homeless" space. In fact, that triggered my imagination, and it still does. The word "homeless" was one we used rarely – except, for me, in a few moments of exasperation.

During these later years, we spent the major holidays together. We would Uber Don to our house or a home where friends were hosting. Every time, he would show up clean-shaven and in tidy clothes, looking terrific – and normal. There was one clue, however, that the person showing up might be homeless or at least home-challenged: a backpack full of dead devices. One Thanksgiving, he inconveniently blew the fuses in the house by charging his electronics, all of them.

These gatherings would end on a heartbreaking note, especially each Christmas. After sharing a lovely time together, we would put Don back into an Uber for the return trip, weighted down with leftovers, gift cards for grocery stores, jackets, and blankets from friends. But there was an ever-present dark feeling, not knowing where he was heading, whether he'd be warm, dry, or safe.

Another example of "normalcy" was our occasional lunches. When he could fit me in, I'd meet him somewhere near where he happened to be living. I was always amazed at how well-read he was. Whether it was the current news or science, he seemed to be on top of everything. Those conversations were no different than other interesting conversations I might have had with anyone, except they were with my brother...who was homeless.

Don was a very proud person. He had a strong ego that we tried to protect by pretending everything was normal. And perhaps this was a way he developed to cope with the life he was living. (In retrospect, it was likely the only way I could cope with the reality that my little brother was homeless.)

Like many of us, my brother had what I came to think of as his personas, a way of acting or a facade that he could switch on and off. When he was with us, he was always himself – the person we'd known before he was homeless. When he came to Christmas dinner, he was Don, my brother. But I suspect that when he left, he switched off that persona and became someone else. To survive. He had the intelligence to put "systems" into place to support his survival. For example, he appeared to have friends in homes where he could shower and wash some clothes.

He had a knack for navigating a lifestyle that worked for him.

Eight months before my brother died, he was diagnosed with leukemia. He spent many of those months in hospitals, ferociously battling the disease. (His years of homelessness and neglect complicated his treatment tremendously, such as extensive deferred dental work had to precede chemotherapy.) But Don wanted to live and was willing to work to make it happen. He formulated many ideas for making the next chapter in his life meaningful for making a difference in the lives of others. It gave me hope that his sense of pride and ability to contribute was intact.

Don received excellent medical care during that time. He was treated with a level of respect by his care team that he likely hadn't experienced for years on the streets. No one knew he was homeless, thanks to his "persona," how he could chat up anyone, and how he conducted himself. And daily visits from family likely also belied his living situation.

Near the end of Don's life, I needed to have surgery. I'm sure he was concerned about me and my health, but he also recognized that my convalescence meant I'd be less able to visit him in the hospital. Two days after my surgery, he called me – an unusual call since it wasn't his habit to phone me unless there was a problem and he needed something. This time, however, he called just to check on me. When I quickly pivoted to him, he said, "No, we're talking about you," which felt genuinely brotherly. The call left me unsettled. His worrying about me was a real role reversal, like having my brother back again.

The following morning, one of Don's nurses – someone I'd developed a relationship with – called, suggesting I get to the hospital as quickly as possible. As I arrived, I heard over the PA system that the patient in my brother's room was "coding." Gratefully, I got to his room just before he died and was able to say "goodbye."

My brother was gone.

Reflecting on Don's life, there is so much I am still taking in and learning. Earlier, I mentioned my brother's sense of self-esteem, his pride, and ego. But if I'm being honest, it wasn't just my brother's self-esteem I wanted to protect through dysfunction and charade. It was my own, as well. Because when I think about who I am and my sense of responsibility to my family, I cannot resolve the dissonance that I knowingly allowed Don to be unhoused during that time.

And yet, I knew my brother wanted to be himself. As tempting as it was to offer free advice and judgments, I knew that, in his own eyes, Don had it covered. At times, I was at my wits' end and terrified for him. According to my own standards, he refused to take the necessary steps to get his life back on track. Once, I yelled at him, "Don't you get it? You're homeless!" I still regret that.

Many narratives flow through my mind to explain my brother's life and how he led it. They range from earning too much money at too early an age, not having to face the consequences associated with an early brush with the law, always knowing he had someone backing him up, being too smart for his own good, and the ravages of drugs. None hold up very well alone. Maybe it's a combination or something else altogether. I'll go to my grave not understanding how the two of us – from the same parents and raised in the same environment – could have traveled such different paths. I'll also go to my grave feeling ashamed and should have done more to bring those paths together.

At the same time, it's impossible not to remember, with gratitude, that no matter how bad things were with Don, he was always proud of me. From attending my election night watch party and celebrating that win to bragging about his sister to the nurses in the hospital, he didn't seem to begrudge our different circumstances. Still, he was always ready to affirm his pride in me.

Don seldom spoke about regrets or sadness and specialized in a philosophy of acceptance: "It is what it is." Yet, when he was at home with my family, I frequently longed for what might have been.

I'll never put his experience in the rear-view mirror. Perhaps because, in a real sense, our life stories are linked. As I consider the profound effect my brother's life has had on mine, I'm reminded that the countless assumptions we make about homelessness are...only assumptions and not answers. Behind each homeless person we see on the streets stands a genuine human being with a childhood, family members who still love them, memories, accomplishments, and dreams. Behind each homeless person, I see glimpses of my brother. And possibly any of us.

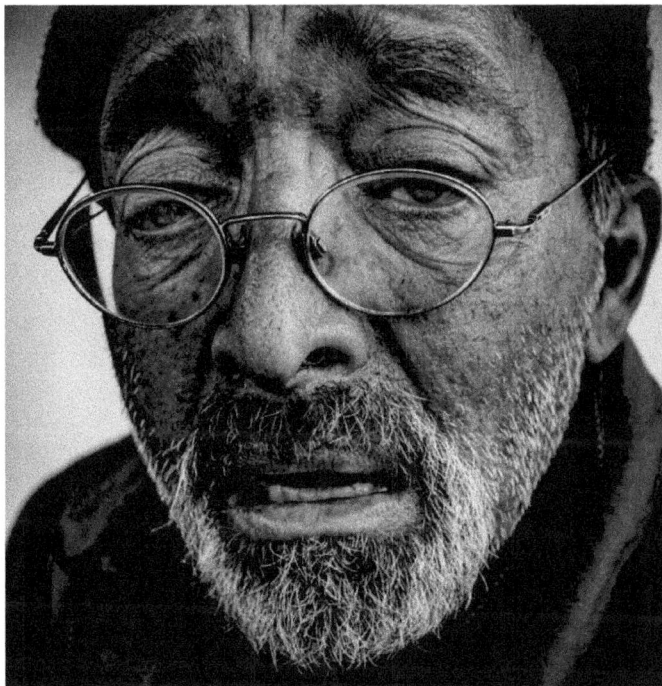

Dignity No Matter What: Collector Edition 2023
Renato Rampolla

Apollo

I spoke with Apollo for about an hour in the shade of a building on the sidewalk as strangers passed.

He said he was once in the Nicaraguan armed forces. He told me times were much different for him at one time as he transitioned from emotional highs to lows during our conversation.

Apollo was not ready to take any steps towards improvement as his drug addiction was overwhelming him.

So much can be construed by the paradigm in which someone believes.

This hit me with a wall of sadness when he said, "I used to have money. I used to be somebody."

Interview with Sister Sally

Tampa, Florida, USA
Hope and Faith: Saved on the Streets

By Dennis Pitocco

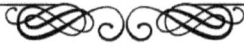

---

*T*he Sunday school teacher held up a picture of people sleeping under pieces of cardboard in a dim alley. "What do they need?" he asked. "Food," someone said. "Money," said another. "Warm clothing," said another. "A safe place," a boy said thoughtfully. Then one girl spoke up: "Hope and faith." She went on to explain; "Hope is expecting good things to happen, and faith is believing in God that they will happen."

They say that faith is work; it's the work you put in behind what you hope and pray will happen. No matter what's happening in the storm of life, it gives you a core foundation upon which to rest, rejuvenate your spirit, and realize not only what's important but how you can use your "gift" of faith to help others. Every story of finding faith on the streets is unique, a tapestry woven from hardship, unexpected kindness, and perhaps a glimmer of hope in the darkest corners.

And that brings me to my encounter with Angela Taylor, commonly referred to as "Sister Sally" (her street name) for the past 20+ years. Why "Sister Sally?" Because she's become the guiding light for those on the streets seeking hope through faith, as you will surmise from my casual conversation ("interview") just outside a local community food pantry where she volunteers several days a week.

Remember, Sister Sally, there's no pressure to share everything at once. Take your time, share what feels comfortable, and know that I'm here to listen without judgment or preconceptions. Your story is unique and deserves to be heard.

How old are you, and where do you live?
I was born in 1970, and I live from house to house. From pole to pole. Helping God's people, the poor, the rich, the drug addicts, the alcoholics.

So, you move around a lot?
From home to home to home, but I never overstay my welcome. I move on when God tells me it's time.

Do people just open their homes?
Yes, sir. They have to trust God to let me in. If you choose God, it's not just about getting a place to sleep but a place to feel safe.

Where did your story of hope, faith, and homelessness begin?
Well, I came to the United States from Jerusalem in 1972 when I was 12. My earliest memory of faith is from the time I was probably about 11. My mom was made aware of some issues regarding my safety that were going on at home. They came out and told her. She said, "Well, I can't just keep her here." So, I was like, "What?" I begged her not to send me away, but she did what God told her to do. And not long after I got here, my family back home in Jerusalem was killed by a local gang.

They had sent me here to live with friends they trusted, hoping and praying that I would have a better life. It was a good life for me. They taught me a lot, like right from wrong, and discipline. They were awesome. They gave me faith as my foundation, which has given me so much strength. I had a bunch of odd jobs over the years, the longest one a part-time job at a local accounting office, but I spent a lot of time wandering the streets, always returning to their home at night. I stayed with them for 18 years until I was 30. That's when God told them that it was time for me to find my way. They put their faith in God that I would be OK on the streets, going from house to house. I knew deep in my heart that it was time to go.

My first couple of nights on the street were scary. I was afraid to fall asleep because the first night, I woke up to some strange man staring at me. I knew I had to come up with a plan. I was on my second day and had not showered or even brushed my teeth. I'm not a fast-food person, but that was the only food I could afford on that day, and I didn't know where else to go. I didn't want to go back to the home I had just left because I didn't think they'd understand my fear since I had God at my side. My vulnerability level was high, and one disappointing word would hurt. Then something hit me like a brick … and I asked myself, "What happened to my faith?"

Things had unraveled so fast for me that I forgot to pray. I wasn't mad at God. I was just confused. But I realized I couldn't hide from God. As the days and weeks passed after that, I found myself practically walking on air with a deep sense of peace and joy. I began talking to and taking an interest in other homeless people who I previously would have crossed the street to avoid. Having no rational, reasonable explanation for my transformation, I concluded that I had experienced a spiritual encounter of the most dramatic kind.

When I first came onto the streets, people were afraid of me because I had a beard and dreds. But I also had my Bible at my side. And then God transformed me, as mentioned earlier. The Holy Spirit was like, you need to clean up your act and help other people on the street find their way. And I said OK, but they need to walk with me and my faith if they really want to change their lives. With a haircut, a shave, and my true self revealed, people who feared me then embraced me. And that's when I became "Sister Sally."

What about the friends you stayed with?
Sadly, those wonderful friends, the only true family I remember, have now passed away. They're gone but not forgotten, as they opened up their hearts to me, gave me hope, and gave me the faith that keeps me going every single day.

Talk to me about your life on the streets today.
You have to know yourself, and then you have to have discernment. You have to have a spirit. So, with me having discernment all my life, if a person comes walking up to me, I can discern them. I was born with that. That's a gift from God. So, I know what they have been through.

I'm so happy here. And I've got friends. God first. And we all look out for each other. We know where to eat, get cleaned up, get personal items, and where it's safe to sleep. I'm lucky because, through the grace of God, I always have a home to sleep in—maybe a different home, but a safe place to be.

Tell me more about "Sister Sally."
I got that name because everyone knows that I walk with God, and they see how happy I am on the street, and they come to me for advice. I try to be an example to them. If they want to pray with me, that's fine. If they want to stop taking drugs or stop drinking, they have to pray with me and accept Jesus as their savior. But if they aren't ready, neither am I to help them. If they are ready, I will take their hand and guide them every day. Some of them have found their faith and found their way into jobs and off the street. Some others have been tested and didn't do well. But I always offer my hand and my heart to those who truly walk beside me with faith.

I never worry about finding food, shelter, or things that I need because God takes care of that for me. And whenever I'm tired or feeling down, I never forget to look up. Because He will guide me; He talks to me. He gives me comfort.

What's it really like to be homeless?
People don't see us. They walk right by. Sometimes, it feels like they are afraid of us. They treat us like we're a bunch of drug addicts and bums who are dangerous. People will step on you, give you dirty looks, make fun of you, degrade you, and call you names for no reason except that you are homeless. People can be hurtful, mean, and cruel. They rarely talk to us or show us any respect. We don't always want money. We just want to be seen.

You have to be very defensive about your things. No matter what you have, someone will want to steal it. You can't store your things anywhere, so you have to carry everything around. Basically, you treat everyone like a potential predator. You hide what little personal belongings you have or keep them on you at all times.

Most of my friends are not here on the street because they want to be. I'm lucky because I feel at home on the streets. And because I'm never alone when God is always with me.

Any final thoughts?
To me, faith is about knowing that this is just one chapter in my life. Yes, sir. There's a lot more good stuff waiting for us. So, I just do what I can every day and hope for the best, not just for me but for all of my friends on the street. And I pray to God that I can help Him save as many as I can.

> *Sister Sally, I'm honored you'd trust me with your story of finding faith and hope on the streets. It's a powerful message. I believe that even in the harshest circumstances, the human spirit can find solace and strength in faith. Sharing your story has the potential to inspire others who face similar challenges, demonstrating that even the darkest streets can lead to unexpected paths of illumination.*
>
> ~ Dennis Pitocco

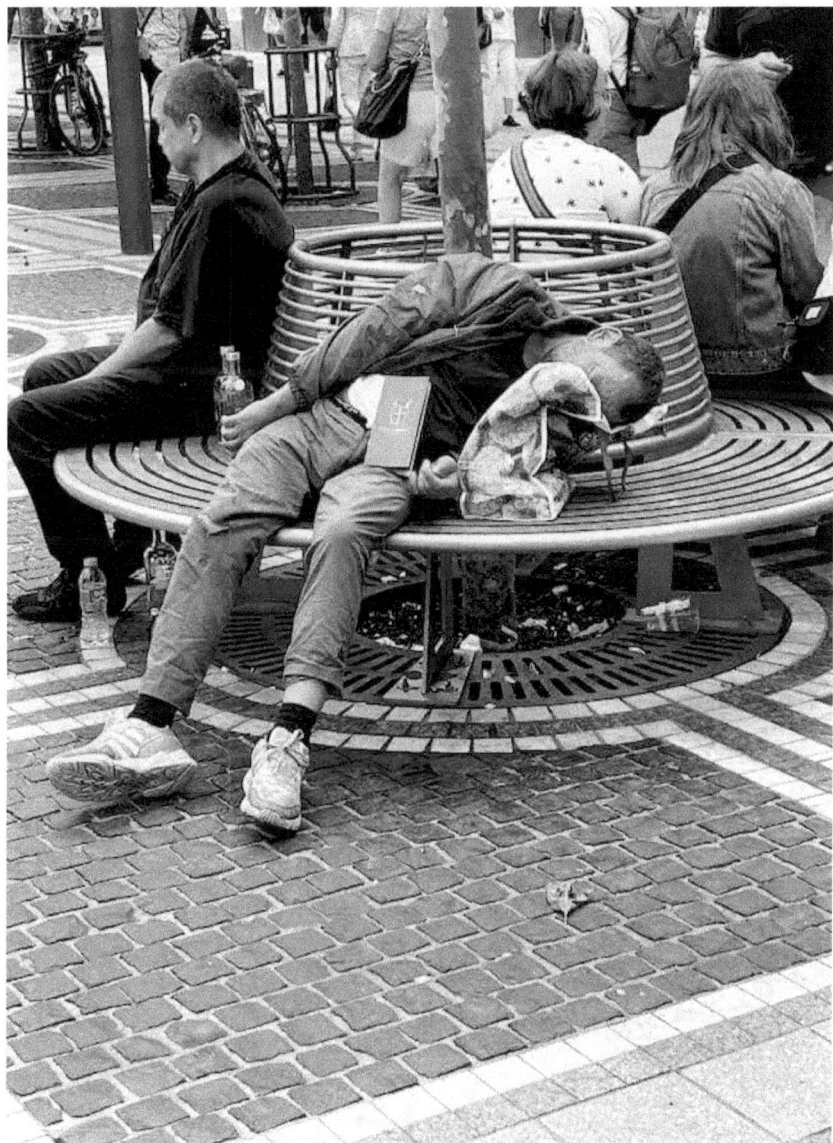

Frankfurt, Germany
Dennis Pitocco, Photographer

A Dandelion's Story

By Brandy M. Miller
Denton, Texas, USA

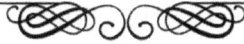

❦❦❦

I loved dandelions as a child. Their bright, cheery yellow heads poking up out of the ground made me smile. I loved the puffballs they turned into during summer and enjoyed plucking them up to blow on them, watching their little white seeds blowing in the wind. It wasn't until I brought my mother a bouquet of dandelions that I discovered the disdain with which other people viewed them. "It's a weed," she explained to me. "Nobody wants weeds."

I knew nothing but love until I was four. Then my father left home and never came back. On that day, I wrote a short story that read, "I am not lovable." Why else would the man who told me he loved me more than anything else in the world leave without looking back? I felt like a dandelion – unwanted, unloved, and discarded as worthless by the man I loved most.

The Impact of a Broken Heart

My heart shattered, and I grew desperate for someone to love me who wouldn't leave me. I accepted abuse and neglect rather than face rejection. I mistreated those who were too nice or kind out of fear that they would learn the truth if they came too close. They would discover whatever it was that made me unlovable and abandon me.

I became a perfectionist because I thought love demanded perfection. Perfection eluded me no matter what I did or how hard I tried. Perfection's tyranny drove me to prove myself good enough for love. The more I did, though, the less loved I felt.

Pregnant, Homeless, and In Despair

My desperation for love drove me to look for love in all the wrong places. I ended up married, pregnant, and homeless at age 19. Those who could take me in wouldn't. Those who would take me in couldn't.

Homelessness felt like leprosy. Nobody wanted you. Absolutely everyone felt it was their right to judge you for being homeless. Nobody cared how you got there. They just assumed you were at fault. I felt so ashamed, and it just cemented my feelings of being unloved and unlovable.

Shelters required us to separate in order to stay in one. I already felt vulnerable. Sacrificing my husband's protection and the comfort of his presence in a hostile world didn't make sense to me.

Getting government help proved a hurdle. The housing wait list was two years long. Because I refused to separate from my husband, the benefits available were limited. I possessed a high school diploma, which worked against me. They prioritized high school dropouts.

We lived in fear of being found by the cops. Each night, we looked for dark places where we could hide the car and sleep for a bit. Trying to sleep in that car in the sweltering Texas heat was beyond miserable. We showered whenever friends would allow us to use their bathroom.

My husband took a full-time job as the overnight shift manager at a fast food restaurant. Once he got his first paycheck, his mother helped us with the deposit, and we were able to get off the streets. The fear of being homeless never left me, though.

At 23, I faced that fear added to a new one: the fear of losing my son. It drove me to a despair so deep I thought about taking my own life. Worse, I thought about taking my son's life with me. I felt like I was drowning in an ocean of problems I didn't know how to solve and wasn't sure solutions existed. No one in my life seemed to live a life free of problems.

It was the thought of taking my son's life that yanked me out of my despair. I decided no matter what it took or how long it took me, I would not quit until I ensured his life would be better than mine.

An Ugly Reality Check

Four years later, I listened, horrified, as my seven-year-old son told me that he was going to kill himself. He explained exactly how he would do it and his backup plan in case that first plan didn't work. This forced me to ask, "What did we do to break our baby to the point that death is preferable to life?"

I didn't know the answer, but I knew I needed to find it. The search for answers led me back to the Catholic Church. I began uncovering the toxic roots of my son's problems, which circled back to the struggles my husband and I experienced with forming deep, lasting connections with others.

In early childhood, I learned that people valued people with money. In my eyes, money made a person worthy of respect and love. I equated money with love.

That's why I set out to become rich when I was four years old. My son's mental health issues forced me to confront an ugly fact: My relentless pursuit of money was killing everything good in my life – including my son.

Prioritizing Relationships over Money

I switched my focus from valuing money to valuing people. I worked on my relationship skills. It was not easy for me to do; those skills take time to develop. The habits of a lifetime are not easy to undo.

I learned new definitions for community with the help of my Church sisters and Worldwide Marriage Encounter. I worked to become part of one. Belonging takes being long in the community past the pain the relationship causes. It requires giving and receiving forgiveness.

As my relationship skills improved, the amount of time we spent homeless decreased. We developed a network of people who knew and cared about us. These people were willing and able to help us through tough times. They remembered what we'd done for them and were willing to repay it when we needed it most.

I reached a significant turning point in 2014 when I published *The Poverty Diaries*. It was the first time I took my past pain and turned it into a tool to raise money to get to my son's boot camp graduation. I couldn't afford to pay rent, let alone afford a 1200-mile round trip for two, but my son's struggles with his mental health returned, and I knew he needed me there.

My experiences were all I could think of to offer in return for people's help. I thought an insider's perspective on poverty might help those interested in the problem understand things better. I left Elko, Nevada, for Ft. Sill, Oklahoma, that August, not knowing how I would get home or if I would have a home to return to. It took us three weeks to make our way back and a little longer to catch up on rent.

A Dandelion's Story

While writing my own story in the spring of 2015, I discovered the power of storytelling and how stories can determine our future. I wrote about the day my father left through the eyes of a little girl and rewrote it as a 40-year-old based on facts the four-year-old me didn't have.

My father felt his paranoid schizophrenia made him a danger to me. My mother agreed. They both believed that he needed to leave for my protection. This changed the story from being about an unlovable girl to a girl so beloved by both her parents that they made whatever sacrifices they thought necessary to protect her. My fear began to resolve itself, and I opened up to love.

That same year, I entered a design competition centered around dandelions and discovered amazing things about them. They are the first food for bees coming out of winter and essential for survival. They pull heavy metal toxins out of the soil wherever they are planted. They assist the body with getting rid of heavy metal toxins, too.

Far from being a weed, their arrival in America came about as a means of helping World War II's working mothers put food on the table.

Their hardy nature meant they could survive almost anything. If there's water down below, a dandelion can grow. Their heads and leaves can be eaten, and their roots can be turned into tea. They are filled with vitamins and minerals of all the right kinds.

Dandelions will grow anywhere. They don't care that other people think they are worthless. They refuse to allow other people's opinions of their value to stop them from bringing good cheer and good value to the world. I decided then and there that I would be a dandelion. I would grow no matter what others thought of me. I would never allow other people's opinions of my value to stop me from bringing good cheer and good value to the world around me.

Dreams and Visions

That December, I set my heart on creating a writer's retreat center. To raise funds, I envisioned developing a reality TV show for writers. I thought it would take $2.5 million to do.

In 2016, I met a woman named Suria Sparks from Singapore. She became my first ghostwriting client. She paid me $3200, the most money I'd ever made on my own products or services. Inspired by my work with her, I wrote and published *7 Steps to Change Your Life & the World*.

I also met the *And I Thought Ladies* that January during a podcast where I pitched my *Writing Reality TV Show* idea for the first time. They became good friends who supported me and encouraged me not to give up.

I worked with many other multi-millionaires that year. I discovered that most of them shared the same struggle. They focused so much of their lives on making money, thinking it would fix their insecurities, that they neglected their relationships. Rather than relieving the insecurities, it amplified them.

They ended up trapped by a life that might look like a dream to most but felt like a nightmare. Isolated and lonely, unsure of the true motivations of the people surrounding them, they feared letting go for fear of who they'd be without the things they'd worked so hard to attain.

Seeing the world through their eyes, I stopped blaming them for the economic situations I faced. I understood that listening to them meant I could learn valuable business and life lessons from them.

Entrepreneurship offered a lot of harsh lessons for me to learn. That August, I ended up homeless again. Right before the crash landing, I met Clara Rufai, Shine Strategist, who needed help with her book. I agreed to help her with her publishing journey.

My relationship skills came to my rescue. I'd mended fences with a man who abused me as a child. He allowed us to stay with him for seven months while we worked to get back on our feet. That's how I avoided being on the streets and continued working with book clients while I got my life back in order.

In 2017, my husband found a job that moved us to Denver, a twenty-year dream come true. We squeaked by financially on his money while I built a business on the side.

In 2018, though, the tides began to shift in my favor. I attended a writing conference in Los Angeles and met several people of influence. One of them was a digital marketing expert by the name of Dima Ermakov, who hired me for copywriting services, and I learned a great deal about digital marketing.

That September, the *And I Thought Ladies* invited me to teach my unique process for fiction editing at an Experienced Writers Retreat in Las Vegas, where I met *Path To Publishing*'s founder and CEO, Joylynn M. Ross. She and I connected and began working together. She mentored me in the business side of publishing.

Turning My Problems Into Profits

In March 2019, I woke up from a dream crying for joy, shouting, "I have problems! I have problems!" God sent me a dream showing me every problem I faced in the past and learned how to solve was today's profit. Every situation I faced but didn't know how to solve was tomorrow's profit. I was never going to run out of problems, but I was never going to run out of opportunities for profits, either.

The *And I Thought Ladies* invited me on a book tour in London in July of 2019. I reached out to Clara Rufai, who I knew lived in the UK, and reconnected with her during my time there. She got me a special radio interview and invited me to speak at her conference in February of 2020. I published *Turning Problems into Profits* in November 2019.

Clara gave me the opportunity to speak on stage in front of an international audience. She also gave me a Creative Strategy award for my book.

Three years later, I developed the *Breaking Open Abundance Program*. It helps others identify and remove the roadblocks to living lives filled with love, hope, and joy. Joylynn beta- tested that program for me.

I came to recognize that the most significant difference between the rich and the poor is not in their bank accounts. It's recognizing what it is they have of value to others. They also know ways to package and present that value - and themselves - to others in a way that makes it unmistakable.

Breaking Open Abundance

My relationship skills allowed me to become an award-winning international speaker and author. They enabled me to co-produce and publish the *Writing Reality TV Show* on a $0 operating budget. Those episodes are all up on YouTube.

I am currently working on a course called *Writing Your Way to a Better Tomorrow*. The course equips others to discover their value right where I once was. In the course, I teach how to mine it, refine it, package it, and present it in a way that makes their value clear.

My main goal for the future is to advocate for all undervalued members of society. The first step is to publish the full details of my story. The second is to build the retreat center so I can help people who don't know their value discover it and build a business around it. The third is to finish my *Surviving the Streets* game. That game will help give people more direct insights into homelessness.

Climbing out of homelessness isn't easy, and escaping poverty is a challenge. I struggle with my finances because I find it difficult to charge others for the wisdom I've gained when I know I can help them avoid what I've been through. Though my bank account remains empty, my heart remains full. I know I'm a dandelion.

After bible study on November 20, 2013, I wrote this poem after listening to people tell me all the reasons that they don't help the homeless.

I Am Homeless

I am homeless, drinking my meals so I don't have to feel the depression and fear.

I am homeless, addicted to drugs that I take to chase away the pain and the tears.

I am homeless, I have no one, no family and friends who will help me out here.

I am homeless, and you chase me from doorways and sidewalks where I stay.

I am homeless, and you won't even let me find rest for an hour or a day.

I am homeless, and you won't hear my story, you're afraid what I'll say.

I am homeless, forgotten, unloved, unwanted, and cold.

I am homeless, the veteran, the addict, the drunkard, the old.

I am homeless, the mother, the child, the abused, the broken, the untold.

I am homeless, there's no room in the inn left for me.

I am homeless, a stranger to a strange land I flee.

I am homeless, sheltering on the ground beneath a tree.

I am Jesus, your savior, in these faces you see.

I am Jesus in the homeless, won't you serve me?

I am Jesus, who gave my life for yours, nailed to a tree.

Brandy Miller ~ *Many thanks to all those individuals along the way who were patient with us and supported us as we strove to make changes in our lives.*

Seeing/Not Seeing

By Cynthia Kosciuczyk
San Diego, California, USA

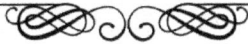

Don't give up.

To set the stage… I am not homeless and never have been. I intend to share only a fraction of my exposure to this population of whom I have compassion and a desire to become part of the solution, not the problem.

I suspect those unhoused feel a fine line between terror and freedom. Though I cannot directly compare my life to those who are homeless, my travel and work experiences have forced me to stretch funds to cover expenses and lean on family and friends for support. The thought of being in a situation with no job, no money, and no food absolutely terrifies me.

After graduating from high school in Worcester, Massachusetts, I went to college and earned my BS in Biochemistry. During this time, I met my ex-husband, a Greek/American. We ultimately moved to Greece to be near his family and friends. I was a Jack of all trades: schoolteacher, worked in the textile industry, and owned and operated a commercial bakery. We intended to stay for a year; it turned into 10.

While in Greece, our marriage dissolved, leaving me to reinvent myself. The following two years took me from Greece to Texas, back to Greece, and ultimately back to Texas. My last Mediterranean hitch made finding work difficult because the island of Rhodes has primarily seasonal work. I worked in a live factory, a good combo for chemistry and cooking. Disheartened by struggling to make ends meet, I was forced to leave Greece for good.

While living overseas, I had little exposure to the homeless. My move to San Diego, unfortunately, changed that. I lived in different neighborhoods in San Diego for the first ten years. I worked in the food industry, which slowly morphed into sales and design. I managed a Persian rug store from 2000 to 2015. The store was in downtown San Diego, where my exposure to the unhoused occurred daily.

From 2018-2023, I moved to a working-class neighborhood and into an affordable studio because of job changes. It had new flooring, was pet-friendly, and was an easy commute to work. When the pandemic hit, many of us were required to stay home for a few months. San Diego's homeless population migrates around the city, a community on the move. Vacant or abandoned buildings are the most attractive. Once their new location becomes populated again, or if they are shooed off by police or residents, they pack up and move on to the next least-populated location.

I became aware of nearby activities because I began spending more time in my new neighborhood. During this time, and much to my surprise, I realized my neighbors were very involved in illegal substances and various other questionable activities. Living close to a shopping mall and a bus line, the alley where I parked began attracting homeless campers. It soon became unsafe. After the office went virtual, a security check occurred daily at 10 PM. Because most crimes and other questionable activities happened after midnight, I began sleeping with the lights on to discourage the crack smokers who liked to gather under my window.

Once we were allowed to physically leave our homes, I returned to the office, but due to the economy, I worked three jobs to make ends meet. Because of my multiple jobs, I was away from home 10-12 hours a day, six to seven days a week. It was nerve-wracking to leave my home unattended during this time.

Surprisingly, not everyone felt this way. There was one resident who frequently traveled, and she kindly opened her home to the elderly who were homeless. As you can imagine, this often escalated into folks being disrespectful and ungrateful.

When my lease was up, I moved to the other side of the building, which, believe it or not, was a completely different experience. I had a view of the pool, not the dumpsters. I felt safer like I had moved to a completely different community. My living space decreased from a 400-square-foot apartment to 275, small but safer.

Though I moved, I continued to be exposed to the homeless population in different ways. My laundromat was only one block away, adjacent to the corner of the Smart and Final, where many homeless people gathered. I occasionally bought an extra breakfast at McDonalds and shared it with those hanging out on the corner. Although the laundromat was well maintained and the owner would be outside in his truck in the mornings, I used the facility at 6:30 AM.

One day, when I went to do my laundry, a man in his 70s – barefoot, wearing only a towel, smoking a cigarette, and clutching a half gallon of vodka – was there. On another occasion, a homeless man was snoring as he slept inside a sleeping bag on the laundromat floor.

I now work north of the city, and my easiest route to work takes me by the homeless camp, making me reflect on the situation. Hardly anyone goes that way as the tents spill into the streets. I have been thinking about the current crisis and wanted to share my experiences with you in this story.

Here is a poem I wrote in 2014.

Seeing/Not Seeing

Walking early morning downtown San Diego Monday

The town on the verge of waking up

Choices: seeing/not seeing

Those whose lives are on the street

Dirty, begging, sleeping
In couples, with pets, handicapped
With carts, with wheelchairs, wagons
All in your face, asking for help.
So, one must adopt a combination of
Seeing/not seeing as one passes by
Just showered, just off the ferry
Walking with purpose to work.
Seeing/not seeing the elderly man
Sprawled on the sidewalk dirty, left leg just a stump
On the sidewalk.
The homeless couple in their sixties huddles under a blanket together,
The crazy one with the wild eyes, all of them looking at me with envy and hope that I
Will have something to share.
Sometimes I see, sometimes I have to not see.

My empathetic heart is pained by life's harshness. I consciously decided to interact with this population instead of judging them or ignoring their existence. When someone was loitering or sleeping outside of our business, and no crime was being committed, I called the bicycle patrol first – not the police. They often knew the person and easily maneuvered them to a more appropriate location.

I learned to keep an eye on the front door. If someone entered, screamed, or became aggressive, I would interact appropriately, asking "Can I help you?" My trained eye watched when their hands were in their pockets. If I felt concerned, I would begin talking on my cell phone and calmly walk them out the door.

I feel the best approach is conversation. Talk, don't touch. They are human, and there is a reason for their circumstances and behavior. My utmost goal was to keep everyone safe and find a solution.

In my personal experience, there are essentially five types of un-housed and various reasons people live on the street.

1. Long-time homeless who "own" their neighborhood
2. Those wanting to argue
3. Those mentally challenged ("The president is going to buy me a hotel. Do you want one?")
4. Ones just needing a place to rest
5. The dangerous kind

Some are not physically, emotionally, or psychologically well. Many simply hit a rough patch in the road, and others have turned to the streets because they find it easier to support their addictions.

For some, the efforts to "fit in" with society can be very stressful. This is especially true for those who have never experienced abundance or kindness; people who have never felt the joys of family or community can feel apprehensive about change. Many veterans also struggle to fit back into society after they return from serving our country.

According to the World Population Review, about 1.5 million veterans are considered at risk of homelessness (being below the poverty level and paying more than 50% of household income on rent). Research shows that the most significant risk factors for homelessness are lack of support and social isolation after discharge. Social networks are significant for those in crisis or need temporary help.

The pandemic has exacerbated the unsheltered populations. Regardless of why someone is homeless, the fast-paced nature of the world and the declining economy are causing people to fall out of the system.

It's a growing concern worldwide, yet I feel it's more prevalent in the USA. Why? When I was overseas, I experienced first-hand how other cultures are more communal, and family, friends, and society more naturally absorb the burden. Food is shared, and there is a sense of inclusion into their community versus exclusion, and there tends to be more compassion for those less fortunate.

Years later, people in my life found it hard to believe I was in such a desperate situation, especially when I returned to the USA. I now have double the space and live in an area where many of my friends live. I work harder to compensate for the cost increase to live in this location. Feeling safe and being able to sleep is worth it.

My heart hopes the world will create a solution that works. As I finish this, I realize it's World Gratitude Day. I'm grateful for having the basics: shelter, food, work, health, transportation, family, and friends.

Hand Up, Not Handout

By Deborah Ling
Sacramento, California, USA

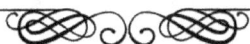

*Though a thousand fall at your side, though ten thousand
are dying around you, these evils will not touch you.*

Psalm 91:7 New Living Translation

I started caretaking for my mom in 2008. She passed away in 2009. I planned to stay in Mom's house by bringing in roommates to help pay the bills and the mortgage.

However, my sister was the executor and refused to allow me to do this. I had to leave the house with no job and nowhere to go—my three years of homelessness at age 54 followed.

Unhoused is the new term, but I was in someone's house for most of the three years, so I did not feel unhoused but homeless. There was no place for me to call home. I did a lot of couch surfing.

Using my laptop, I searched daily for a job and submitted my résumé to anyone hiring. My résumé at that time was quite impressive. I had been the owner of two businesses and one nonprofit and an office manager in two jobs. I had managed an air conditioning and heating company with 20 technicians. Scheduling them daily was no small feat during the summer in Southern California! In another job I had, there were 15 maintenance technicians. I created a preventive maintenance program, which saved the company a lot of money.

Unfortunately, only fast-food places were hiring at this time, and they would not give me the time of day. I was so overqualified. When Christmas rolled around, I thought I would get a job, at least for the season—no such luck. No one would even interview me, let alone hire me.

The first place I stayed after my mom passed was with a gal I volunteered with. As long as I could pay her, I was welcome.

**But when my money ran out,
so did the welcome mat.**

Another time, I rented from a guy who was renting the house. There were several of us; most were seniors. One day, he packed up and left us all high and dry. He failed to pay the rent with the money we had given him, and he shut off the electricity, literally leaving us in the dark. We had nowhere to go, so we stayed there and did our best until the day the sheriff showed up. They gave us one hour to pack our things and leave the house. We packed up and placed our things in the yard, unaware of where to go.

After this event, a couple asked me if I wanted to sleep on their couch. I had nothing to lose, so I jumped at it. I only stayed there for about a month after I realized the guy was selling drugs. Being as straight as an arrow, it freaked me out. But I did not know what to do other than to keep looking for work to help get myself out of the hole and praying for my protection.

One day, the guy came and told me they needed me to leave. His customers thought I was recording them when I was on the computer when they came to make a buy. He said besides, he was expecting the DEA to raid his house at any time, and he did not want me there when that happened. Well, I couldn't argue with that! I got out of there.

In between couch surfing, I was in two different shelters. The first one had two buildings. One building was for single women, and the other building had families. Some were couples, some were single moms, and the rest were single dads. They had to have children in order to qualify for this shelter. The program required daily chores and to attend to their classes.

In the classes, they would help you write up a résumé or teach you how to interview. They taught us what employers were looking for. Then they showed us the door and told us to find work.

The shelter was not in an area with many stores, which required us to take a bus to look for a job. That took money, which many of us did not have. The shelter did not provide a connection between what they told us we had to know about getting a job and actually finding one. It was a total disconnect. After 90 days, I was told to leave.

I did not understand this at all. Other women had been in the shelter when I arrived, and they were not being told to leave. It was not fair that other women got to stay longer than 90 days. I contacted the director, but the conversation was fruitless. But at least I got it off my chest.

After I left this shelter, I ended up walking around downtown. I connected with a few others who were also homeless. I thought I would be safer with other people. That night, we stayed under an awning. It rained all night. One of the guys I was with got drunk. He had a knife and told us he would slit our throats while we slept. One of the other guys told me not to worry because he would ensure I was safe. I was cold, wet, and scared.

**The only thing I could do was pray
for the Lord to keep me safe.**

The next day, a Navigator (one who works for Sacramento helping the homeless) saw me. She asked, "You do not belong on the street, do you?" I burst into tears and responded, "Noooo." She took me to a house shelter operated by a church.

The house shelter had three bedrooms. One room was for the monitor, one had three beds for men, and the other had two beds for women.

I had only been there a day or two, and one night, while watching TV, I smelled bleach. I just figured someone was cleaning, and I continued. Later, when I went to the bedroom and opened the door, I gagged. The smell of bleach was so strong I could not breathe. Even though the other girl was already in bed, I turned on the light to find out why I smelled bleach. All of my clothes and books were covered with bleach.

I called the house monitor and got him out of bed to show him the problem. He called his boss and told him what had happened. Then he told the other girl she would have to leave in the morning for what she had done. He returned to his room.

Being allergic to bleach, I had difficulty breathing, so I threw my stuff in the garbage and got everything out of the room. I then pulled back my covers and found that bleach had also been poured onto my bed! I called the house monitor back into my room. That was the last straw. He told her to pack up and get out. I had to sleep on the couch for three days while waiting for a new bed. I was there for 90 days.

I also stayed upstairs in a church for a while. There was little privacy, as anyone could come upstairs at any time. I never knew when someone would come up those stairs. There was no shower, so I had to sponge bathe. At least while I was there, I knew I was safe.

Finally, I found work through an online site and was hired as an editor for someone writing a book. I had been editing for about twenty years, showing my experience in that arena. When one project finished, I looked for another one. I built up my profile to become one of their top earners.

Now that I had an income, I could start looking for a place of my own to live. However, I found I was not making enough money to rent an apartment, so I decided to rent a room. Even though the owners of the two homes I rented were very nice, I was uncomfortable using their kitchens. I felt like I was intruding on their family. So, I would purchase microwavable food, allowing me less time in their kitchen. I am still friends with one of the landlords.

I was finally able to get
a one-bedroom apartment through HUD.

For obvious reasons, living in the shelters, a church, on the street, and in others' homes is uncomfortable. I had to swallow my pride, accept handouts, and live in places I would not have otherwise. I am grateful that I was not on the street for long and had a roof over my head most of the time. Some places I stayed could have ended worse than they did. I am so glad they did not. It was enough of a nightmare as it was.

I understand how humbling this type of life can be and how hard it is to keep your self-respect. I despise how people treat the homeless, who are down and out. Many want a hand up instead of a handout. Those are the ones I want to help.

Deborah Ling ~ *What got me through it all was my faith. I trusted the Lord to keep me safe*

Interview with Kaylee

Conroe, Texas, USA
By Lynn Forrester Pitocco

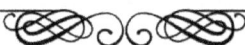

Truly I tell you, whatever you did for one of the least of these brothers and sisters of mine, you did for me.

Matthew 25: 40-45

*I*n my lifetime, I have had moments of close contact with those who are homeless. Many strive to return to normalcy: a roof over their head, a hot shower, and a place to cook a meal. However, in one of my conversations with a homeless man and woman, I also realized that some choose to exclude themselves from society.

In many towns and cities around the world, dead souls are plastered along our streets and highways. In some impoverished cultures, a lack of housing and a job ignites this unfortunate outcome. In other cases, it is often a result of an unexpected chain of events.

When we see someone standing on a corner holding a sign: "Anything will help," "Hungry," "Homeless," etc. What can or should we do? Do we stop and hand out a few pennies? Do we strike up a conversation? Do we hope we are not the first car in line when the light turns red? What do we think as we wait silently for the green light?

I recently interviewed a young single mother, Kaylee. I reached out to her through channels I have through our church. I inquired how I could help her obtain items for the girls. Kaylee agreed to the interview because she wants others to learn from her story.

Kaylee has three young daughters, ages six, five, and three. Growing up, Kaylee's home life was dysfunctional; her stepdad was an alcoholic, and her biological mother had schizophrenia, bipolar disorder, and was a drug user. At the age of nine, Kaylee entered foster care. Though her mother was unable to take care of her, she would not allow Kaylee to be adopted.

While in foster care, Kaylee attended school and did quite well. Though she graduated from high school, she began using drugs and alcohol her senior year. With no transportation of her own, she relied on friends for transportation. After graduation, she continued to use alcohol. She was unable to hold down a steady job, and her mother totally detached from Kaylee due to bipolar episodes. Kaylee "aged out" of the foster care system and found herself on the streets. By the time she was 23, she had three children; none of the fathers were a part of the children's lives.

Kaylee suffered from postpartum depression after the birth of her first daughter and continued drinking in excess, causing her to become an alcoholic. Kaylee lived in an old beat-up car and stayed in and out of hotels as she tried desperately to keep Child Protective Services at bay. She finally established conditions allowing them to stay together but never owned a house. An Uber driver sexually assaulted Kaylee at age 20, and her youngest daughter was a result of that sexual assault. Through the help of friends, Kaylee never lost custody of her children.

Kaylee began using a social app called "Next Door." Next Door is a platform where you can discover your neighbor-hood and connect with people in the community. At first, it was difficult; people were not willing to help. She continued to post comments diligently, and ultimately, people were willing to support her financially.

Her younger half-brother, age 16, lived with her briefly until he was brought into juvenile court for truancy. With their mother's medical condition, she was unable to care for him and ensure he went to school.

In the last month, Kaylee has found an apartment through the Montgomery County Women's Center. The center maintains support for women with children in need of shelter. But she can only stay there for 18 months and will have to move out. She works multiple jobs, cleaning, running errands, organizing, etc. Unfortunately, Kaylee's mom is out of the picture entirely, and she has no relationship with her father or grandparents.

Kaylee, what do you fear the most?
"Not being a good mom for my girls. I never, ever, never ever want to be homeless again. I now feel safe. I want to provide a good home, a stable home for me and my girls. Being homeless wasn't what I wanted, and once you are there and alone, climbing out of this situation is difficult."

After all that you have experienced, what is your wish for the future?
"I have been sober for four years. I want my daughters to grow up healthy, and I want to have my own home someday. Though I feel safe where we are currently, we are not out of the woods yet, but I am determined to keep us off the streets."

When I reflect on the worldwide homelessness issues, I wonder how those of us who are fortunate to have the basics in life can step up and work collectively to stunt the growth of this epidemic. Might we become more empathic and compassionate for those who have encountered hardships, trials, abandonment, and neglect by society and, in some cases, their own family? Acknowledging and listening to those in these unfortunate situations increases our understanding and allows us to work together to help get men, women, and families off the street.

As I circle back to my conversation with Kaylee, I realize we can all make a marked difference in finding solutions to reduce this epidemic, even if we just begin by listening.

Lynn Forrester Pitocco ~ *In my life, as a single mother, I have encountered being on the verge of homelessness, having little money to sustain a simple meal for my young daughter, standing in line at food pantries, sleeping in my car, no gas for my car, yet; without warning, a simple soul senses my situation and without asking extends a helping hand. Perhaps an angel in disguise without a name that I never got. Thank you!*

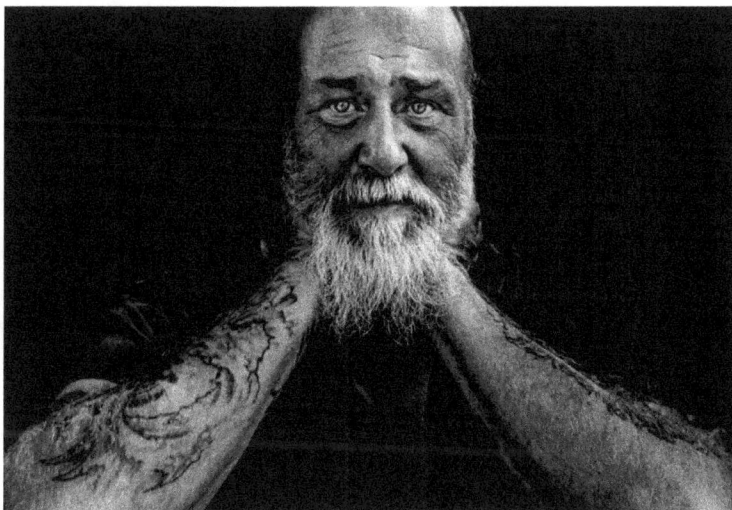

Dignity No Matter What: Collector Edition 2023
Renato Rampolla

Beau

Often people who live outdoors congregate in "self-made homeless camps" on vacant lots that have plenty of shrubs. In the South, they use fishing line to tie together palm fronds for privacy. Cooking and heat is usually rendered with Sterno because the smoke of a campfire would bring attention to their location.

Humans are social creatures, but more than that, grouping together is a way of protection. It seems almost every week, a person who lives outdoors is beaten up, knifed, or shot.

Tattoos are prevalent and often made by other people in the groups with staples. Tattooed on Jim's left bicep is a hinge in the open position. This tattoo is sacred to him as it reminds him of his state of mind when he used to inject heroin in his arm each day...he said he would become unhinged. In the screw holes of the hinge are the exact locations he inserted the needle that provided his daily heroin fix.

He has an infectious smile and converses easily about his past. I could see him as a salesman or businessman. He's charismatic and quick-witted.

"I'm not addicted to that s*** anymore!"

"What's that you're lighting up?"

Spice. You wanna hit?"

Broken Treasures

By Andi Buerger, J.D.
Redmond, Oregon, USA

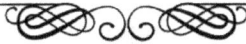

*The heart has its reasons of which
reason knows nothing.*

Blaise Pascal

Home.

That's a powerful word. Powerful in that it conjures up common images of a tangible dwelling where one or more persons might live, celebrate holidays, or host others for meals and fellowship. In this way, the power is in the fact that people with a physical address or location to call "home" feel more secure, confident, and accepted by others in their circle of influence, regardless of the value of the structure. When there are multiple homes in a neighborhood, there is the power of community – an inferred support system resulting from owning or renting a home in such a neighborhood.

Home is a powerful word for other reasons: When a person lacks a physical address, permanent residence, or tangible shelter, the lack of a home works against them on a larger scale. There is no community for support during hard times when someone is unsheltered. Often, there is unwarranted judgment about the person or family on the street or in a temporary shelter. While those without a home may be employed, earning respect is challenging without a physical residence someone can see, visit, or assess at tax time.

When was the last time you encountered someone on a street corner, in a thrift store, maybe even at church who did not have a place to sleep or live? Were you curious as to why that person was homeless? Did you ask why they lacked the means or resources to provide themselves or their family with a motel, trailer, or other secure shelter? Maybe it was easier to presume their homelessness was due to alcoholism, drug addiction, mental illness, or even criminal circumstances.

Judgment is always easier than verifying facts or truth.

It takes less time to judge someone and, in many cases, eases the conscience of the one judging because they can smugly go home to a warm dwelling, food in the pantry, running water, and clean sheets on a real bed. Arrogant disregard for personal firsthand knowledge only fosters the continuance of situations such as homelessness. I know this because adults taught me that people *deserved* to be on the street because they had done something "wrong" in their lives or made bad decisions. If I didn't want to become *just like them*, I needed to finish school, attend college, and get the proverbial "good job" to ensure my general safety and societal acceptance.

It would be decades later before I learned firsthand that not every unsheltered person had made decisions so poorly that they deserved public disdain and dismissal as valuable members of communities.

Many were shattered treasures with pieces of worth strewn across years of hardships, grief, troubled relationships, challenging illnesses, other personal adversity, and even discrimination. Those unsheltered were – and still are, to a great degree – *broken treasures.*

This I know. I, too, was a *broken treasure.*

In 2008, I experienced my fourth massive brain injury out of nine, which affected my ability to continue my work as a highly paid corporate trainer. The loss of income (and a year of memory) impacted me on many levels. With this pivotal life-changing moment, I could easily have ended up like many other out-of-work and unemployable people due to my injuries. Add to that my own traumatic experience of being sexually abused and trafficked – long before there ever was a term called human trafficking – from the age of six months to 17 years old by family members; I knew I had to find something else I could do to serve others.

So, my husband Ed and I established Beulah's Place, a 501(c)3 nonprofit that has provided temporary shelter services to at-risk homeless teens for fourteen years. We saw a need in our Central Oregon community to help teens living in cars, parks, and occasionally couches from Good Samaritans – sometimes without their knowledge! By designing a temporary safehouse system with a three-to-five-month timeline per "guest," we were hugely blessed to rescue and assist over three hundred teens in our area, plus a few outside of Oregon.

Each guest was required to sign a binding contract outlining expectations and non-negotiable requirements, such as completing high school and acquiring and maintaining viable employment, to participate in our program. The housing was graciously provided by volunteer host families who were properly vetted. They often became repeat host families due to their experience helping an unsheltered teen "graduate" into successful independent living in their community of choice.

The reintegration of these young adults meant that they required little to no assistance during their first year after graduation from Beulah's Place. Twelve of the adult teens we rescued have now completed college, thanks to the generosity of donors and host families. One of our rescued teens was legally adopted as a young adult. It was a landmark moment for my husband and me to become "official" parents the day we adopted Allison.*

Allison had called Beulah's Place just two days after her eighteenth birthday. Her father had sexually violated Allison from a very young age, and her birth mother was too busy with alcohol and a boyfriend to protect and nurture her. Leaving six frozen dinners in the freezer for Allison each week, her birth mother left her to fill her own needs every week from the time Allison was age twelve to seventeen years old. The mother only came home when Allision tried to commit suicide on two occasions. When Allison called our shelter, she was unwanted, unfed, and unsheltered as a teen. If *only* for Allison, everything Ed and I sacrificed personally to keep Beulah's Place going and to rescue as many youth off the streets as possible was totally worth it. No regrets.

*Each year, an estimated **4.2 million** youth and young adults experience homelessness in the United States, 700,000 of which are unaccompanied minors – meaning they are not part of a family or accompanied by a parent or guardian.*[18]

As the safe house hosts and I worked with the teens, including a few boys who were brave enough to ask for help, one overriding pattern emerged: why they were unsheltered and untethered to any family system. The pattern was that of *permitted* sexual abuse by a parent or partner of a parent. The *permission* refers to the fact that the abuse was known or reported to one parent or adult, but nothing was done to protect the child or children involved. Additionally, parental negligence, instability, or flat-out abandonment of their teen began long before the teen took to the streets, hoping to escape the cycle that drove them out in the first place.

Once on the streets, every teen we rescued or interceded for admitted that the streets were not "friendly" to new arrivals. A pretty young girl, Evelyn*, knew she was at risk the longer she stayed on the streets. Each night, she would walk around our town as soon as it got dark and didn't stop until daylight. Now and then, a friend would let her climb through an open window after the mother had gone to work so Evelyn could clean up and nap before hitting the streets again. As Evelyn told me during our meet-and-greet interview before placing her in a safe house, "I heard

---

[18] *NCSL (March 29, 2023)*

people on the streets were like a family. They watched out for each other, but that's not true. It's a hard place to be. People are mean and only look out for themselves."

Like Evelyn, most people she encountered on the streets also came from a world of hurt and pain. Some had mental health needs that went unaddressed. For various reasons, others simply couldn't keep a job long enough to sustain regular housing. *Someone* had to help. *Someone* had to intercede for the ones who did not choose the circumstances that drove them to unsafe environments and lack of safe shelter.

Every 40 seconds, there is a child abducted in the United States.[19]

It is a myth that every teen on the street is a runaway – the falsehood must be exposed! Otherwise, our nation will continue to lose its future and its hope – our children. While there is a small percentage of youth who choose to run away, my decades of working with teens and young adults who have been trafficked by sexual predators and victimized have taught me that most youth find themselves in these situations without any provocation on their part. All in all, discarded and abandoned by those who should love and protect them.

Myth-mongers are the *real* barrier to finding solutions and preventing unsheltered youth.

Forty-eight hours is the window for a teen that has "disappeared" or gone missing before he or she will be approached or taken directly into a human trafficking situation, primarily sex trafficking. Since most law enforcement agencies require a twenty-four-hour waiting period, that leaves one day for action to begin in the search.

---

[19] David Washington, Director of the U.S. Marshals (2020)

What happens to a teen who applies for a summer job in your neighborhood but finds out the ad posted was not what it seemed to be? Shopping malls are notorious feeding grounds for criminal predators. Yet, thousands of teens every day get lost in the throng of shoppers, vendors, and those looking for unaccompanied or unaware victims.

We need to be more diligent as parents, guardians, and community partners in protecting all our children by having age-appropriate conversations about human trafficking and also what life "on the streets" can be like for the teens who see it as a solution to their perspective on mom and dad's rules and restrictions at home – whatever that home looks and feels like.

For the teens and young adults who do end up unsheltered through no fault of their own, the risk of assault, sexual violation, abduction, and other violence that could lead to their death is exponentially increased. Many people in my city had proposed creating a shelter system for unsheltered adults and families. Prejudices and biases kept "something like that" from being discussed thoroughly, let alone built.

The popular reaction from those I spoke to on and off for nearly fifteen years was along the lines of "Nobody wants a shelter with criminals or addicts in their neighborhood or around their businesses, Andi."

I wondered if these folks had ever visited a well-operated, friendly community shelter where structure and compassion go hand-in-hand, residents are provided the tools and resources needed to fit their specific situation and timeframe, not just the standard "food and bed" for just a day, but maybe a week or a month. Feeding and bedding the homeless is absolutely necessary, but is it enough to help someone change the course of their current circumstances?

After a decade, Beulah's Place was able to purchase a 4,000-square-foot building that had been abandoned and needed tens of thousands of dollars in repairs to make it usable as an extended day shelter for teens. The plan was to reduce the number of suicides in ages 14-21, increase regular attendance in school, offer free tutoring, assist with job skills and viable employment, address medical and dental needs, and provide dedicated "rest zones" where weary bodies could sleep even for a few hours (since we were not zoned for overnight care), and include the resources on site that identified and addressed to the best of our ability any addiction or mental health concerns.

This unused school district building had not been utilized for many years, stood across from the city offices and parking lot, and sat on the corner of an older neighborhood.

Generous contractors and others lent a hand to repair and refurbish the building, and it wasn't long before a neighborhood petition was passed to block our use of the building for a teen shelter. The woman leading the action had never spoken to me, asked any questions of our volunteers, and never visited City Hall to verify we had a permit to operate as intended.

While one neighbor did take the time to speak to me during a fundraiser in the parking lot of our building, his questions represented that universal myth about anyone in a shelter. "So, you're not going to house criminals here? They're not juvenile delinquents?" No, and no again.

Post-pandemic and with the current state leadership at that time, many nonprofits serving communities struggled with reduced donations and funding. Our lender felt the pinch, and suddenly, Beulah's Place was forced into selling the building as quickly as possible. My husband and I had been covering costs here and there over the years, especially as more and more teens entered our program, but we could not continue covering the mortgage on the building. The interest alone was around $1,400 a month.

Human nature is, well, human nature. After the building sold, I received a curious email from a business owner in town. She had "heard" that we had a shelter for a "bunch of teens," and, as a landlord in the area of that building, she was concerned about property values. In very diplomatic terms, I informed the business owner that she had been given incorrect information. We hadn't owned that building for over *two years*.

*Your branches will be home for many
searching souls as you grant to those who mourn in Zion,
consolation for their souls.*

Isaiah 61:3

Every person who enters a shelter has a story. Whether they are a one-time guest or become a "regular resident" of such facilities, how can we genuinely serve the needs of the unsheltered if we don't know who they really are? We must dig deeper into individual needs rather than assigning one generic "homeless" label to them to successfully release unsheltered persons from repetitive returns to a system versus some form of home.

Communities, in general, need to create forums or opportunities on a regular basis to have conversations publicly that are respectful, compassionately moderated, recorded, and then addressed within a specific timeframe, with results published for all members to see and hear. Bring experts, shelter directors, and – yes – a variety of unsheltered individuals and families willing to speak about their experiences and who may have valuable perspectives to share.

Statistics show what is reported or allowed to be reported. Thousands and thousands of "hidden homeless" live among us. Those persons may couch surf or live with others temporarily because they have no permanent housing available. Young people often make up a large percentage of the hidden homeless because they have had some crisis, trauma, or other change that precipitated their unfortunate situation. While the term "affordable housing" sounds good from a podium or platform, waves of these projects claim to be affordable for those less fortunate in their communities. The reality is that many are not affordable at all – not for the minimum wage earner, a family where two parents work full or part-time, or even families who "combine" themselves under one roof to pay the rent or mortgage and avoid becoming homeless.

One of the young women my shelter rescued now has two toddlers. Her family's small affordable housing rent is $1,400+ per month, without utilities, diapers, daycare, and more. With the rise in food and gas costs, feeding three mouths plus traveling to and from work and daycare centers landed this family in their car for a period of time. They are now housed again, but for how long?

In the U.S., I have witnessed how the economic and housing crisis has sent families and children to the streets because they can't afford rent, let alone buy a home. The choice is to move on to an area that may offer lower living costs, but will work be available in that new location? Do children have to start over in new schools? What human costs are involved where "affordable housing" isn't affordable?

A friend of mine had to leave our area despite having a professional job that paid well, with benefits to boot. She simply couldn't afford the ever-increasing rents for a small condo in a despicable condition, which the property management company was not anxious to address. Her rent was the equivalent of what a mortgage for a high-end home in our area used to be just a few years ago!

Now imagine a single person, an elderly couple perhaps with health issues, an adult teen, and others all looking for a place that represents *home* to them, whether it be an apartment (also rent prohibitive), a trailer, a tiny home, or another secure structure, every human being needs a safe place to rest their head, to escape the pressures of the world, and – if they choose – to raise a family safely.

In the absence of a home, unsheltered programs are a good first effort. Food, hot coffee, a cot, and a decent restroom are better than the alternative. When Beulah's Place began, we addressed "basic needs" until we understood each of those teens' stories and underlying needs.

Like branches of a tree, my husband and I saw the opportunity to bring young, unsheltered souls searching for consolation and a chance to find a future and hope into a community willing to receive them. Every life is a treasure in God's eyes. Every heartbeat has value. While some have experienced great brokenness and despair, there is always one place where each of us can feel our full worth, reach our potential, and shine like a priceless jewel.

It is a forever home…it is God's heart.
And there is room in His heart for every human being.

As they say, "When one chapter closes, another opens." Before Beulah's Place closed, God woke me up in the middle of the night and nudged me (hard!). "More voices. Get 'more voices.'" I could not get that concept out of my mind or heart. The giftings He gave me would allow a larger net to be cast and save thousands more, maybe millions, down the road. His inspired name was *"Voices Against Trafficking* (VAT)."

Now, through God's amazing grace only, VAT will address victims of child abuse and sexual exploitation, plus tangentially related human rights issues such as hunger and homelessness. VAT has a magazine called *Voices of Courage,* an upcoming TV show of the same title in 2024, and two books on Amazon.com with a third coming out in early 2024, a global music fundraiser project ("CD fundraiser" for short), one educational and two safety and prevention curricula first launching in the U.S. and a special "recovery house" pilot we hope to put in every state.

We also have two special skills teams ready to execute live rescue and relocation missions once we have funding in the next 6-12 months from the CD fundraiser and other domains and sponsorships. The music compilation project will be available on CD, flash drive, and digital download. It was released in November 2023 with Public Service Announcements (PSAs) recorded in 31 languages! All this in less than five years.

Do not pass a hand in need,
for you may be the hand of God to him.

Proverbs 3:27

Andi Buerger *~ Dedicated to the courageous hearts of those innocents I was honored to rescue and assist in helping them find the future and the hope they deserved. The unconditional love of God given to me was poured into their indomitable spirits making them the overcomers they always were, but just didn't know.*

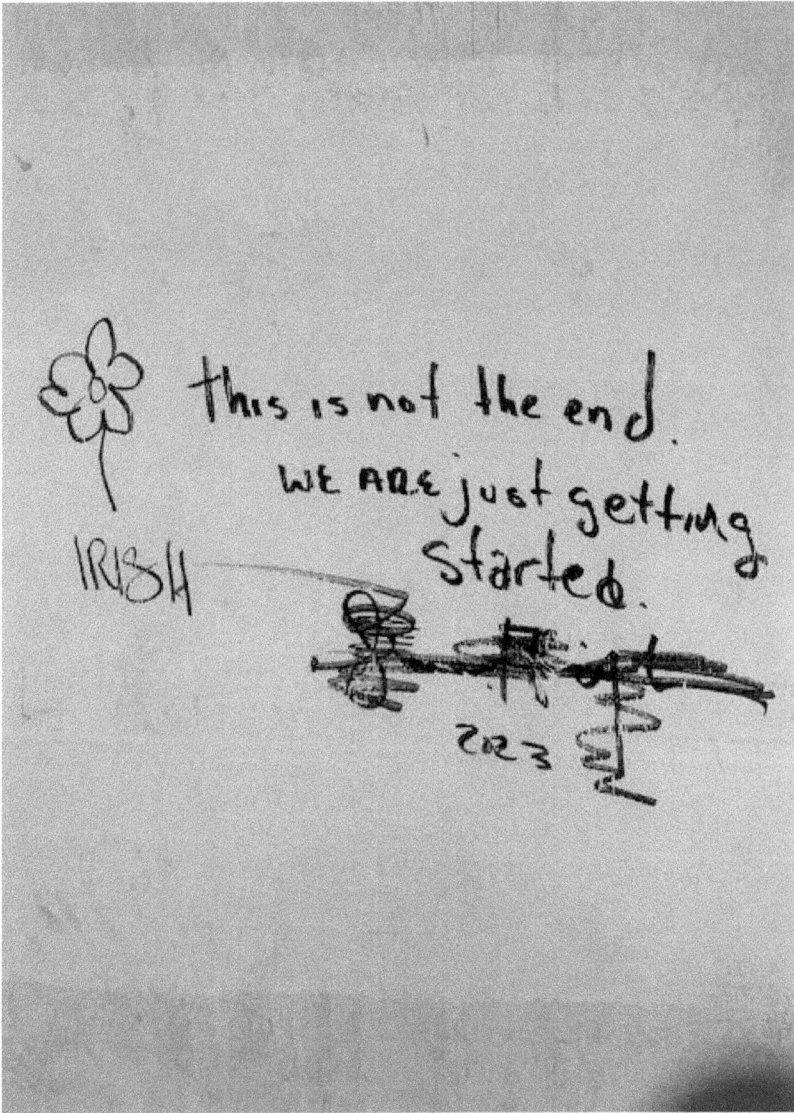

Graffiti Las Vegas, Nevada
Dennis Pitocco, Photographer

The Difference

By Joseph Carrabis
Northern Maine to Mississippi

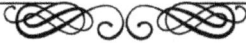

Ful wys is he that can himselven knowe!

Chaucer, The Canterbury Tales,
The Monk's Tale

*T*here is a difference between sleeping in the cold because it's an exhilarating wilderness experience and because no warm place will have you.

There's a difference between sleeping with your three-month-old son on your chest because it's a loving, bonding experience and because you're sleeping in your car and because it's the only way to keep him warm in the harsh northern New England winters.

There's a difference between dumpster diving because it's a frat kick and because it's the only way to find food for your family.

There's a difference between having doors closed because there's no room at the inn and being slammed in your face because people don't want you near them.

There's a difference between waking up soaked and frozen because your fever broke and you're on your way to health and because your son pissed through his diaper while he slept on your chest in your freezing car, and you don't have another one for him to wear.

There's a difference between standing over an inner-city sewer grate because you're imitating Marilyn Monroe and because you hope the rising steam will keep you warm for one more night.

There's a difference between not eating for a week because you're fasting for health or political reasons and because you're not eating means your wife and son can.

There's a difference between eating raw corn for its nutritional properties and because it's the only thing you could steal from the farmer's fields before he loosed his dogs on you.

There's a difference between abandoning your family because you don't care about them anymore and because you know they will be taken in and cared for once you're no longer with them.

There's a difference between being beaten as part of some training or as an initiation rite and being beaten because people fear your presence will somehow contaminate them.

There's a difference between self-hate and self-love, and I weep for those who have only learned the former and don't know how to learn the latter.

There is a difference between where I was some sixty years ago and where I am now. But every time I sit in my car on a cold winter's night, waiting for the engine's waste heat to fill the passenger compartment, to clear the windows, to stop my breath from steaming, my son's ghost sleeps on my chest, his urine runs down my sides, soaks my shirt, and I reach for another rag that is not there, to cover him, dry him, keep him warm, and I weep.

The Story Behind The Difference

How did you become homeless?

I became homeless because all other doors either wouldn't open or were slammed in my face, hence I had nowhere to go except the street. My other option was suicide - something I'd already failed at three times – and homelessness seemed the best option at the time.

Why were you turned away and not helped?

You'd have to ask those who turned me away and didn't help me. Let me also offer that phrasing the question as "Why were you..." infers blame and responsibility on the individual being addressed. Asking "why..." is, in English and many Western European languages, called a "defensible" question, meaning it places the addressee in a victim frame by asking them to defend/explain their actions and reasonings with the hidden reference being some kind of judgment by a supposed superior/authority figure. Ask someone "why...," and the sympathetic nervous system and amygdala go into overdrive. People's blood pressure rises, their respirations change, their facial tonus shifts, ... And it doesn't matter if the exchange is friendly or not.

Top-level psych workers are taught never to ask "why" questions. It's a useful tool in interrogations, sometimes in negotiations, rarely, if ever, in therapy.

How long were you homeless?

Any length of time without basic security/safety is too long. I lacked any form of security or safety from childhood through my early thirties.

How did you turn it all around?

With great effort and lots of work. If there's another way, I wish I knew it then and would love to learn it now. Despite everything I experienced growing up, I repeatedly and confusingly scored off the charts in intelligence and similar tests. Confusion ruled because I had extreme difficulty learning anything. Dyslexia was unknown; neurodivergency (a term which amuses me on many levels) was unheard of, and although I was blind, no one took that into consideration except to mock, bully, or otherwise humiliate me.

I could also solve the most intricate math, physics, and engineering problems with no effort, while textbook questions bewildered me. I could sit with a family of non-English speakers for half a day and speak their language without an accent, but learning French in a classroom left me deaf and dumb (an unpopular term now, *de riguere* in my youth). Any successes I had in life were deemed flukes, accidents, chance occurrences, or due to the intervention of others because I was considered incapable of manifesting success on my own.

In my early thirties and during an act of road rage (as documented in my novel, *The Shaman*), I stopped, suddenly aware that acting out (a metaphor of acting irrationally and perhaps violently due to psycho-emotive issues) was not how I was supposed to live my life and also aware I was not controlling my life.

The Universe was watching out for me because, seeking help, it paired me with an amazing and brilliant therapist (who I modeled my own work after). I told him once that I felt if someone were to open me up, to really get inside me psychologically, they would face a nuclear explosion, so great was my suppressed rage, and I asked more than once if he could hypnotize me under restraint (a life of hard physical labor made me extremely strong for my size) to learn what I kept holding back.

As we got closer and closer to my core issues (sexual, physical, mental, emotional, and spiritual abuse from about the age of three to twelve/thirteen, followed by all except sexual abuse until I was in my early twenties), my rebellion became more intense, and I asked if he could commit me to a psychiatric hospital.

He did, and there I met another brilliant gentleman, this one the hospital's chief psychiatrist, who was another gift of the Universe to me. Together, these two individuals showed me respect and trust – amazingly brave of them, considering my history.

I remember taking an R-PAS while there. There were some images to which I shook my head and said, "Next." At the end of the series, I said, "Let's go back and get those I missed."

The psychiatrist administering the test stared at me for a moment. "I've never had anyone ask to go back if they missed an image."

I returned her gaze. "You think I want to be this way? Don't you think I want to be well?"

The chief psychiatrist later told me everyone was impressed when told this. When it came time to part with my principal therapist, he shared how amazed he was at the amount of work I did to heal. "Most people can't escape a past like yours."

I pay tribute to that therapist and the chief psychiatrist in the dedication sections to several of my books.

Since that time, I've studied and published in over 120 different fields, created a base, disruptive technology that was adopted worldwide, and early on made a conscious decision to help others similarly "gifted" (and more of this later). But my greatest joy? Both asked me to join them in their practices after I started researching and developing techniques to help people similarly afflicted.

How did this affect you and your family long term?
My family of origin considered my situation par for the course; how could it be any different? I was Joseph after all, and everything happening to me was my fault; nobody else was to blame. During that time, a beautiful woman made the horrible mistake of marrying me, and we had a son.

It was during this time I started manifesting my father's behaviors. A "rageaholic," my father would routinely beat me with a rubber hose to the point of unconsciousness (mine, not his). If not the hose, his fists (I clearly remember him boxing me into a kitchen corner because I spilled some dishwashing soap in the sink).

I never struck my wife or son, and the fear of becoming my father – I knew no other way to parent – caused me to bring them to my mother-in-law's home and essentially abandon them there. As I wrote in…

The Weight:

So, one day, I asked if she'd like to go down and visit her mother in Virginia. Her mother hadn't seen the baby, so that seemed like a good idea.

"Let's stay a couple of weeks. Give me a chance to see if there's a good job down there."

I think she knew. She must have. How could she not know?

The third day there, I told her I was going out for a pack of cigarettes. She looked at me for a minute but said nothing. Finally, she just kissed me and let me go.

I don't know why I said that. I've never smoked cigarettes.

I didn't know how to save myself and would not allow myself to behave to my then-wife and son as my parents and other relatives had behaved towards me.

Have you shared with others how this experience affected you then and how it still haunts you now?
Read the first part of this entry for an idea of the haunting. I started sharing my experiences in writing groups. I was insulted, reviled, verbally abused, and told to leave, which I did, thank goodness. My writing could never have matured otherwise. Since then my books, stories, and poetry are routinely cited and honored by readers, reviewers, and other authors.

Do you work with or support those who have found themselves in your past situation?
My self-examination and education led to my being invited to be one of the first members of the New York Academy of Science-United Nations "Scientists Without Borders" program. Modeled after *Médecins Sans Frontières*, participants went where needed to aid others. In 2010, I was invited to become an International Ambassador for Psychological Science. The Nature Group also invited me to represent them at some international conferences.

My self-work led me to develop different methods and techniques for helping others with PTSD deal with their situations. Rejected initially, those methods and techniques are now part of the literature, and I've trained psych-social workers internationally in their use.

Perhaps my crowning success is the response to my *The Augmented Man*, a novel in which I wrote about many of the techniques and methods I developed and demonstrated their use. I've had enumerable people email, write, message, and otherwise reach out to me to share how much the book has helped them in their own lives or their family situation. Psych-social workers repeatedly contact me to let me know the novel's "Through" section is a handbook for dealing with people working out of trauma.

Personally, I spend time each month in volunteer activities aiding those who live as I lived. Principally, I let them know they are heard, seen, accepted, witnessed, honored, respected, valued, and loved.

My greatest gift, me thinks, is letting them know they are loved. This is a lesson I learned from my previous dog. He shared with me once that being warm, safe, fed, and dry are wonderful things to be thankful for.

But if one isn't loved, they are nothing.

Joseph Carrabis ~ *Thanks to everyone who made this necessary.*

Shi(f)t Happens

By Lonnee Rey
Boulder & Denver, Colorado; Maui, Hawaii;
Seattle, Washington; Las Vegas, Nevada, USA

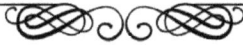

It's not what you look at that matters; it's what you see.

Henry David Thoreau

*D*uring a commercial break, Tyra Banks leaned in, took my hand, and said, "You are so brave to do this." The syndicated show had never done a live swab test for HIV. Eyes wide, I glanced at the front row full of counselors seated nearby to "catch us" if we "lost it." As guests, we all had good reasons for needing a test, and Tyra was doing it with us for the show on guarding your personal safety: three beauty pageant winners and me. I thought, *Nah, I'm just a dumbass who lived to tell about it, literally.*

I said, "Tyra, my biggest prayer was, 'God, make this matter someday. *Surely,* I'm not going through this @#$! for nothing, even if that means I'm the poster child for what not to do.' "

"Mommy! Look at that lady's arms." I was skinnier than Olive Oyl, and embarrassed to be seen. By the time I was on Tyra Banks, I'd been homeless a few times already.

Sometimes, we end up in places,
doing unexpected things...

"Yeah, ok, I guess you can stay here. You can sleep behind the sofa and keep your stuff back there with you," Mike said. I was never so grateful for a roof over my head. It's too bad I didn't think of that during all those days when I didn't work, or couldn't work, because I'd been up for three days partying.

I'll never forget riding my bike to the food bank in a snowstorm in Boulder, CO. It was either do that or wait a week to pick up my food box. The bus wasn't an option: it required two quarters. Lint was the only thing lining my pockets. The woman with so much going for her lost it all in a puff of smoke.

Eventually, the local homeless shelter had an opening, and I got a real bed. A favor from a friend helped me get a real job. The "stay" is limited, and once again, I got lucky: I fell in love with another "resident." He seemed really serious about changing his life, too. We moved out of the shelter and into an apartment together. I was hopeful that life took a turn for the better. Then came the day I heard, "Hey, Miss Lady, he's using again and sharing needles." Wait, what? Needles?? That was news to me. Oh crap. The dream of "coming up together" became a nightmare in seconds.

You can't possibly know how discouraging it is to try to do better but fail, fall, and fumble the ball repeatedly. Despite my Pippi Longstocking life of adventures, much of life has felt that way. It's hard to keep going, hanging on to a shred of hope that things will get better…that someday this will make sense, or matter somehow, to someone, somewhere, God help me.

Things did get better. Angels in pants (friends, boyfriends, total strangers) appeared out of nowhere to help me with a home or a job, sometimes, both in one. Sadly, I screwed it up every single time.

I'll never forget the night I had to escape my own home when a fight broke out. Quickly packing a small wheelie suitcase, I jumped out of my bedroom window and ran away with a guy I really liked. I thought we could "come up together" no matter what just happened. But the place he took me to was a drug den. A snarling old woman yelled, "Give me back *my* suitcase!" She took it from me, opened it, and went through my things – what little I had left. "Leave her alone! She's an innocent," someone else shouted.

I have no idea why that stopped the invader, but it did. Gathering my things, I quickly left, alone. Thank you, Shouting Angel. Roaming the streets was better than a drug den, but I was exhausted.

"Get UP! Get UP NOW!"
A stranger was standing over me.

"You cannot sit here in this parking lot crying like that! Get UP, or the police will take you away. WALK. MOVE. KEEP MOVING. Las Vegas police don't give a damn how you got here, and you don't want them taking you to jail over it. GET UP!" Thank you, Move It Angel. I walked, sobbing my heart out, all night long.

Whether wandering the streets or trying to stay hidden, walking the alleys instead, there have been angels who appeared out of nowhere to guide me to safety, offering shelter for the night.

Commiserating with other down-on-their-luck kinfolk felt good, yet inevitably led to a "spot" for the night...or five. Common sense says, "Get away. Find new friends. Change your ways." Yep, all good ideas, but the reality is, in the light of day, it is damn near impossible to climb out of that black hole.

With each backslide, I sat on the ground a bit longer than the time before, wondering, "What's the use? Why bother getting up? How did this happen? *God, why am I going through this?*" I can't tell you how many times I wished for my own death.

Ten years before, in search of meaning and a reason for all the angst, I'd sought the help of an amateur birth chart reading group. Six people huddled over my printout. Eventually, they called me back to the card table.

"We just wanted to see if we are on the right track. We see here that you were three years old when your parents divorced. Is that right?" Holy crap. Yes.

"Wait, hold on here," I said. "You can see an event involving three people on *my* birth chart? Is it all there? Is it all already done??"

The spokesman hesitated as he said, "Well, there is free will."

"Uh-huh. Ye olde fallback, free will. Let me ask you this: What if I make a left-hand turn instead of a right-hand turn? It may look like free will to me, but wouldn't that moment also be on the chart?"

He never answered. We both left with a lot to think about.

None of us know what another person's blueprint says, so how can we begin to know that person's journey?

And what about karma? As the ghostwriter of *Kicking Karma's Ass* (2022), researching the topic was part of my job. I wanted to address the definitions and beliefs about it. Was it really my client's bad karma that brought on so many tragedies? Or was it hers to live through, "spinning hay into gold," as she put it, so her story would someday serve others? With *"Unbelievable stories of strength, resilience, and perseverance, all told with a twist of humor"* as the tagline, it ends well and is slated to be made into an inspiring movie.

Whether her trials were karmic, none of us can say for sure. Looking in from the outside hardly gives the whole picture of what's going on for someone. Sadly, my client dealt with a ton of haters as if her life wasn't bad enough already.

**While it's true that we shouldn't care
what people think, we do, if only because
their judgmentalism is an invisible barb.**

It stings, so we all try to avoid looking too outlandish lest the people talk. Otherwise, I'm pretty sure everyone would wear pajamas to work. But we don't; there are societal regulations few dare to breach. No wonder Cos-Play events are so popular: creative clothing and full-on self-expression are fun as hell when everybody is doing it. But as fun as these events are, they are not "normal."

Is "normal" the only way to live? Who says so?

"Two arms, two legs, no excuse not to be working," my brother said. "And anybody who chooses to live outside is crazy."

Hmmm. "The homeless population in Knoxville, TN, increased 50% between 2020-2021. There is no way that we suddenly have a rash of lazy or crazy people," I said.

Coincidentally, 2021 was also the year Knoxville declared homelessness a felony. The process: arrested, held for three days, and fined $3,000. All but two states, Oregon and Wyoming, have made homelessness illegal. That fine is ridiculous enough, but finding work to pay it off is job-hunting on a whole new level. Life after a felony is full of limitations. A felon cannot apply for certain housing assistance programs, either. It varies by state. Dang, that's a pretty steep penalty – for life.

I said, "Does it really matter how people end up without house keys if the end result is the same? In your eyes, is one reason better than another? This brings up a deeper question: Without asking someone directly, how do you even begin to guess their side of the story in your head? This happens IRL: In real life, people are so quick to assume rather than ask, then judge accordingly, casting slant-eyed looks and cold barbs at the unsuspecting soul. Isn't it bad enough that soul is on the ground already – must you kick him as well?" My brother had nothing to say.

It is hardly a fair shake, but that happens all too often. It totally sucks being on the receiving end of misunderstandings or worse, bald-faced lies repeated by malcontents. You've been there; you know how it feels to be rejected by people who don't know you – haters whose emotional narratives are supported by other half-lidded beings – none of which give two rat's asses why, how, or what happened to you.

To ask, you would likely deflate their overblown sense of ego and snuff out their righteous indignation. In other words, it'd be a buzz kill to have compassion...to see that maybe, just maybe, shi(f)t happens without much notice.

When a friend invited me to live w/her on Maui, I bounced. It was the first time I'd moved on a one-way ticket where a friend was waiting on the other end. I say this because every other time, I leaped into the void solo. It always worked out. Even so, her presence didn't help much.

Without wheels, Maui is a hard place to be. It limits your job options to live-in jobs. Being dependent on other people, subject to their whims, can be nerve-racking as hell. You're in a spot: theirs. If it goes sideways, you're o-u-t, or you stay, feeling compromised. That happened to me as a live-in nanny. I stood up for the kids, and it quickly went downhill from there.

As usual, somehow, my "next" worked out. I met the right person, who happened to have a shack available on his off-grid property. The organic farm I landed in was a gift from the gods. My "Little House on the Prairie" lifestyle dream manifested in the nick of time. Feeding the chickens was the highlight of my day, and carving chopsticks in the shapes of my fingers by lamp light was nighttime good times. As the domestic goddess, it worked out. We ate better, and even our common space sparkled with three inches of dirt gone.

And then came the news that I needed to fly back to Seattle for a deposition. A minor car accident left me with a major whiplash, and we were finally going to court over it. Tossing my bag into the Yellow Cab, and with one foot inside the taxi, the secondary property owner said, "Eric invited you, and he isn't here. He's in Greece. I'm not grandfathering anyone in farming, so you gotta go. Don't come back. Have your girlfriend pack up your hut and ship it; I don't care. Just don't come back."

And there you go, literally…in a flash, I was homeless. What happened then? Obviously, I made it, but the details are foggy, frankly. The point is how fast your bottom can bottom out.

In *Rattled Awake: Volume Five*, my chapter, "Peace of Mind," was written with "Don't be scared, be prepared" in mind. Several oh-shit events prove how the acts of others can destroy one's reality faster than you can say "Jack Flash." For instance, the 10-alarm fire that left dozens of residents standing outside, shivering, as the blaze engulfed their reality. The ones who had insurance easily moved on to stay in hotels. The remaining residents were left to figure it out. Not only did they lose everything, but they were also starting over with how it ended: barefoot, in pajamas.

**Shi(f)t happens to the best of us.
Sometimes, through no fault of our own.**

Little did I know that the day I responded to a Craig's List ad, "Have you been putting off getting an HIV test? National talk show host wants to hear your story," would become an answer to my prayer that someday all of this would matter to someone, somehow.

As I wrapped my arm around Tyra's waist, we closed the show with a deep bow. Sheer terror turned into a sheepish grin: the HIV tests were negative. That day, at least, it all made sense.

I'd lived to tell about it, literally, once again.

In 2008, the only work I could find was daily-pay temp labor. The 4-hour gigs didn't net much. Homelessness was staring me right in the face, once again. I look back now and laugh at how panic-stricken I was, even as I type these words. It has always worked out. Duh. Still fogging a mirror...

In the thick of it, though? Man, it's hard to remember that somehow, it always worked out.

One night, I said, "God help me!!" It was a "depths of my being" kinda desperate, you know? THAT'S rock bottom. I *really* meant it: "God, *help* me!"

As if on cue, I swear to God, my landline rang. My head said, "The labor force people don't call at night about working the next day. Who the hell has my number?" My gut said to answer it.

You know those long pauses on the phone, where you just know a telemarketer is about to say something? It was like that – I was ready to bail.

The caller begged me not to hang up on him. I knew that voice. "WHAT do YOU want?!"

He said, "I've been looking for you for 10 years. I can't believe I found you."

"Yeah, well, I told you we were done. It took a long time to get rid of you. And you still tracked me down?" I was pissed. "WHAT do you want?"

"I need you to come to fix my practice again. Before you answer, I'm calling from Australia. I moved the practice down here a few years ago. I really need your help."

Depending on how I looked at it, this choice sucked. Working with a man who still pines for you gets messy quickly, especially with *him*, or staying in God-awful Denver and expecting The Crash of '08 to take me down.

A peculiar man, the Aussies didn't like him one bit. Cue "shock face." I hated to depend on anyone, *especially* him. He could make a nun swear. Trying to rebuild from nothing often equates to such compromises, though.

The Mixed Blessing Angel sent me a way out—a lifeline, right on time. In five days, I had a one-way ticket to Queensland, Australia. Soon, I grew his Chiropractic Bio Physics practice in a country I never imagined visiting. It was incredible. Challenging, yes, but it was a leg-up out of the cycle of homelessness. Whew.

Thank God, shi(f)t happens.

Lonnee's Personal Affirmation: *I AM divinely guided, connected, and protected.*

Homeless Among the Stars

By Earth O. Jallow
Ohio, USA

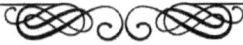

*B*uzz, buzz, buzz. The sound of my phone brought me out of my sleep. I had turned it on silent earlier because I didn't want it to wake Erykah.

I slid the phone from under the pillow where I lay on her tour bus guest bed. The caller ID showed it was Koya, my best friend. While I was traveling on Erykah's *Mama's Gun* tour as a magazine journalist for *Urban Flava* Magazine, Koya was looking after my girls, one in elementary school and the other a toddler.

Urban Flava magazine debuted its first cover with R&B hitmaker Eric Benet, and from there, we were on the map in the music industry. *Urban Flava* was blowing up the celebrity scene with fresh interviews, reviews, and A-list talents like Rakim, Erykah, Jill Scott, and more. And I was thrilled to be a journalist for the magazine. We worked years on this publication, built it from scratch, and it was finally about to start paying us back. I had landed my first big gig.

Worried that something may have happened to my girls, I answered the call. "Hello?" I whispered into the phone, trying not to wake Erykah.

Nothing could prepare me for what Koya said next. "Hey, sis. I hope y'all made it to Canada safely. I didn't want to call you earlier with this, but when I went to get the girls' clothes, G was packing your stuff. He said he'd gotten a storage unit for it and was putting you out of the house."

Her voice sounded defeated. I heard her but still heard myself saying, "What?!"

She started to repeat herself, but I cut her off. "Wait! Are you serious?"

"Yes. He said he didn't want you there anymore. What are you gonna do?"

In shock, I began crying into the pillow.

There wasn't a damn thing that I could do from another country. Being homeless with two young daughters was never in my plans. I couldn't, and I wouldn't mention this to anyone on this trip. I didn't want to get kicked off the tour. Adding missed opportunities and unrealized dreams to homelessness would equal hopelessness to me, and I didn't need that ugly lifelong disappointment sitting on my shoulders, breathing down my neck, for the rest of my life. I had to stand strong for my babies, so, "What am I going to do, Koya?"

Koya replied, "I can ask my Aunt Tara if I can keep your girls at her place until you get back. Then we can see what happens when you pull back into Ohio."

My mind reeled from the shock. What else could I do but accept her offer? What did I do to deserve to be put onto the cold streets with my children in winter? Why didn't my roommate tell me his plans before I left? Was it because I'd turned down his sexual advances?

I'd saved a little money while living with him, but not enough to cover first and last month's rent on a new place, plus all the items the girls and I would need to move at the last minute. I still faced the inevitable hurdles from owing back rent and late fees to the prior apartment complex.

"That's cool, Koya. Thank you for having my back. I'll call you tomorrow when I have some private time. Erykah is sleeping in the bed, right next to me, and I don't want to wake her with this nonsense." Tears and snot ran down my face.

"Ok. Stop crying. There is nothing you can do about this now. The girls will be cared for, and God's got the rest! Get as many exclusive interviews as possible and try to enjoy some of the trip. We will talk tomorrow. Good night." The phone went silent.

This trip should have marked the start of my dream life of being a celebrity journalist. Instead, it marked the beginning of my silent nightmare of living homeless among the stars.

I was a young, single Black female start-up entrepreneur with two daughters, living in a city with no blood family nearby. My stability wavered quite often, leaving me scared and lonely. I formed bonds with people I met along the way, hoping our philosophies aligned: morals, values, human decency, and love towards their fellow man or woman.

But sometimes, people are good actors and slip under the barbed-wired fence we build around ourselves. You never see the destruction coming, even while sitting in the front row of a theatrical production of your life.

Caution: Proceed with caution; the signs flash, but we ignore the warnings and trust others with our basic needs and safety and those of our loved ones.

These are the times that we must take responsibility for the choices we've made.

My roommate was a drummer from our dance company and a platonic friend with two young sons of his own. Six months back, I shared I was struggling with my apartment costs. He agreed to help the girls and me by allowing us to move in with him and the boys.

We would do the communal living thing and help one another with the children and their activities since I was just getting started with journalism. I would pay him a fraction of my previous rent, allowing me to play catch-up with my old apartment complex on the back rent. Everything seemed to be working out and looking up for us.

Then that call came. I kept my mouth shut about my problems and dove into the tour at full capacity to keep my mind off my children and our situation. I not only interviewed everyone in Erykah's entourage but every celebrity who gave me so much as a fleeting glance. I even played nanny to her first son when her personal assistant was busy with other duties. At one of the stops, I was asked to announce to the concertgoers the women who were on that leg of the tour. That city had an all-woman lineup, and I was the woman they got for the job.

Every night was a different city. Every day, I was closer to returning to Ohio, but I had no idea what I would return to other than the disappointed looks on my daughters' faces.

One morning, I was eating breakfast with Erykah and her son. He was crying at the table. It was nothing serious, just a toddler being fussy. Erykah said to him, "Why are you crying? Do you know how blessed we are? Save those tears for magical moments. This, son, is not one of them."

At that moment, I decided I would not cry about my situation one more time. Nothing about being homeless was magical to me. I also wanted to save my tears for something magical, like my comeback.

As the tour bus rolled along the highway, like the thoughts in my head, I knew I would soon face real-life problems. Erykah sat in the middle of her tour bus bed, listening to tunes that, once again, I'd never heard before. She looked so beautiful doing what she loved…music. She was very graceful, gracious, and kind to let me travel with her, her son, and her band family, share her space, and eat with her. She shared her soul with me, but I couldn't do the same. She would never know the depths of my gratitude as the homeless journalist on her Mama's Gun tour.

As the bus pulled into its final stop on this leg of the tour, I wrapped up the prayer I recited silently and glanced out the window at the Philly nightlife. The sign on the building read *The Electric Factory*. This is where all the stars do their big concerts in Philly, and I was here tonight to witness a few. Musiq Soul Child, Jill Scott, The Roots, and Talib Kweli were on the ticket, along with Erykah. It was my last night living out of hotels and tour buses. My last night eating whatever I wanted.

My last night knowing where I would lay my head.

Koya was there to pick me up from the Columbus Airport. "Hey, Sis, how you doing?" she asked with a smile.

"Why are you so happy knowing I'm homeless, girl?" I asked with my head tilted, lifting the suitcase into the trunk of her Honda.

"Girl, I told Aunt Tara what happened. She said you and the girls can stay with her until you get another place. How much time do you think you will need?"

I was silent for a few minutes. I wanted to give a reasonable and truthful answer, but I was unsure.

"I think two to three months should do it," I said. "I have a few dollars saved up, so I should only need about three more months to feel secure."

I pray that's all I need, I thought.

As the car bobbed and weaved through traffic, I could feel my anxiety kicking in as we sped towards Aunt Tara's house, somewhere I'd never been before.

"Tomorrow, can we go to the storage unit so I can grab some clothes? The only items I have are the clothes in my suitcase."

"Sure, Sis, I said I got you!" Koya said. I believed she meant it. *Thank You, God, for sending a real friend in my time of despair.*

We arrived at Aunt Tara's place with its brown door and green awning shining under the light of the winter moon. Koya pulled into a parking spot. She popped the trunk and headed to unlock the door to my new "normal," at least for the next several months. I remained at the trunk, just standing there, looking at my single lonely suitcase and my laptop bag. At that moment, those were all the material possessions I had. I sighed deeply and closed the trunk—time to meet Aunt Tara.

Once we got the girls off to school and daycare, it was time to head over to the storage unit that contained my life. I had been pretty quiet for the last twenty-four hours as I processed the tour, my girls, and the situation of being a homeless Black woman with two small children.

**Once again, circumstances forced me
to place my trust in others.**

We drove up to the "U Store It" facility and entered the security code my ex-roommate gave me through texts. I didn't have any desire to see him at this point.

We drove to the back of the storage facility, and before Koya dug the key out of her jacket pocket to unlock the unit, my stomach began churning as my anxiety kicked up. As I heard the click and before Koya lifted the thin metal, all the breath left my body.

My eyes could not believe what they were seeing. All my things were literally thrown into the space. It looked as if he stood outside the unit and pitched each item, including the girls' bunk beds. I froze in place, staring at my life turned upside down. I felt small, unseen, uncared for, and unloved.

As I stood there with hot tears streaming down my cold cheeks, I felt a snap inside of me, and I broke down to my knees. "Don't cry, Sis. Get up off the ground. It's cold out here. I know you're hurt, but I promise you will be OK."

I responded, "I was cool until now, but seeing how he just threw my things in here like this is beyond disrespectful and cruel. I'm hurt and don't know if I will ever forgive him for this!"

After digging for clothing for the girls and myself, we left the unit with the few items I could find. A calm came over me as we returned to Aunt Tara's place. It was a feeling that felt hot, rising from my feet and slowly climbing up to the top of my head.

Never Give More of Yourself than You Can Afford to Lose.

Earthizm

I knew at that moment that I would be just fine. It might not be today or tomorrow, but I knew just as sure as the sun was shining on that cold winter day my life would eventually be exactly what I made it with the love of my daughters and my new best friends, Koya and her Aunt Tara, the Guardian Angels that God sent in to assist me in my time of extreme need.

That's how I learned that you can have it all together on the outside while your world is falling apart internally. I might have been a fresh journalist who landed a gig traveling with A-list celebrities, but I didn't have a place to live in real life. Homelessness doesn't mean you live on the streets; it means you don't have a lease with your name on it. And I was homeless among the stars.

Earth Jallow ~ *Thank God for keeping me in a standing position when so many times all I really wanted to do was buckle and fall. My daughters, Marquesa and Yacobia, Brandy Miller, Joylynn M. Ross, Koya Howard, and Aunt Tara...I Love Y'all!*

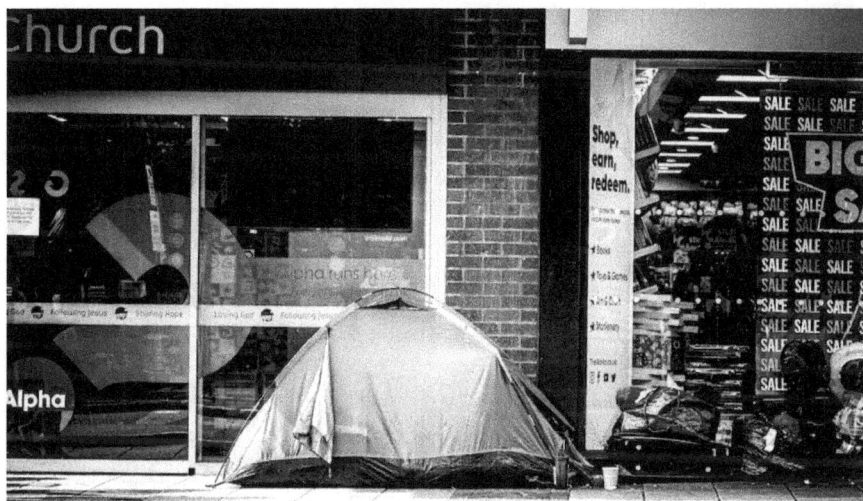

United Kingdom
Sarah Harvey, Photographer

Unhoused by Choice

By Jack Everly
Germany, Spain, Sri Lanka, Thailand, Australia,
Oakland, California, and Boston, Massachusetts, USA

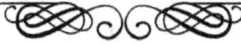

───── ⌾⌾⌾⌾⌾ ─────

Kindness calms the severest of storms.

Jack Everly

*A*fter seven grueling but ultimately rewarding years as a Pilates studio owners, my wife needed a change.

She decided to close up shop and travel the world. Always committing to doing things right, without shortcuts, we spent May, June, and most of July 2018 selling or disposing of our not-100%-necessary thingamajigs, doodads, and trappings.

Goodbye to Carmelo[20], the bright, banana-colored Fiat that served me so well. Likewise to Skeletor and Skeletoria, the two happy-go-lucky, glow-in-the-dark toy skeletons hanging from Carmelo's rearview mirror. Goodbye to furniture, appliances, music- and videocassettes, DVDs, CDs, five pairs of shoes, ten pairs of underwear, twenty pairs of socks, and my whoopie cushions (alas!).

Not only adults made the hard choices; our youngest child, who would accompany us as well, was forced to ask which toys, dolls, and clothes

---

[20] Car-Melo-Yello; get it?

she should take and which she should bid adieu. Princess Goldlily, the My Little Pony with the stupefyingly annoying voice? A shoo-in for the trash heap, but what about the three-foot-tall stuffed Rabbit, Winnie the Pooh's "friend," who kept her company from her first waking moments?

Other people often remarked how they would like to travel, and we echoed such desires ourselves. We both agreed, however, that doing it was a lot more fun than talking about it, and so, giddy to a fault, we embarked.

We've since traveled to many corners of this world. We've seen five continents and been around the globe at least twice, depending on how you measure it. Being out and about gives one a deep appreciation for freedom and the ability to move untethered from one place to another.

Of course, traveling has its downsides as well...

TOP TEN DISADVANTAGES OF TRAVELING

1. You WILL visit some hygienically-questionable toilets. For some reason, I recall a story[21] from Southeast Asia about a man crouching over a squatty-potty and being bitten on his Bangkok by a gargantuan python. It didn't happen to us, but still...

2. With your worldly goods stuffed into colossal backpacks, maneuvering through airports and crowds is exhausting. Also, my petite wife, so encumbered, resembles some kind of mutant turtle. At least our efforts in the studio granted us strong backs.

3. One man's potato soup is another's...not. Our decade-long vegetarian/vegan lifestyle enabled us to often forget that many, if not most, people enjoy their soup with bacon bits. Likewise, Lamb's lettuce. Finding healthy, unprocessed meals fitting our peculiar diet proved to be a Herculean task.

4. Old careers do not translate to success online. Beverage delivery had no future on the web. Further, new habits are difficult to

---

[21] https://www.bbc.com/news/world-asia-36394819

develop, and Fiverr makes millionaires of no one I know of – at least not writers.

5. Mopeds are dangerous. They do not handle well on sand. 'Nuff said?

6. This world is a beautiful, rewarding place, where "This world," however, should be understood as "Nature." And I list this as a disadvantage because although we are fully aware of Nature's unspeakable beauty and utility, it's impossible to enjoy any of it without green. No, not grass. Entrance tickets to America's glorious National Parks are pricey indeed. Those who need Nature's healing and restorative powers, the poor and traumatized, never get by the gate.

7. Speaking of money, Australia is expensive. So is California. The rest of the planet is swiftly catching up.

8. Airports have little respect for humanity. Period.

9. You come into contact with The Unfortunates. On a beach in southeast Sri Lanka, an alcohol-reeking, middle-aged man revealed to us without prompting that the tsunami of 2004 took ten members of his family. We stood exactly where the Wave made landfall. And speaking of the woeful:

10. Nary a day will pass when you do not witness someone living on the street.

The problem is ubiquitous, so much so that we were both forced to wonder where the problem comes from and why it's so hard to remedy. In our studio, we often had customers who suffered because of this injury or that chronic condition, and it was my wife's job to decipher the cause of these maladies so the person could then put it behind them. This end result would have been unreachable had my wife not looked at and understood this cause.

Homelessness arose with the first cities, I'm guessing, but achieved "national issue" status in America in the 1870s. England, however, has dealt with the matter for an eternity. Authorities jailed vagabonds under the Poor Laws of 1383. In the sixteenth century, they spent three days and nights in the stocks. In 1530, lawmakers introduced whipping as a solution to the pesky problem without effect. Seventeen years later, another law subjected vagrants to two years of servitude and branding with a "V."

As first offenders, BTW. Death resulted after a second offense.

Still the concern persisted into the 1700s, when, out of desperation perhaps, English policymakers shipped hordes of ramblers off to America. Out of sight, out of mind [wipes hands clean]. Yes, many of America's founders descended from vagrants or their sons and daughters.

The facts disturbed my wife and me, but inevitable trips to subways and bus stations, even airports around the globe, gave the problem faces and names. The one-time issue of homeless humans had become a plague.

When the Stock Market crashed in 1929, Herbert Hoover responded by blaming the Mexicans and forcing one million of them back to their original homeland. Somehow, the Depression continued leaving two million homeless people to migrate across America and stay in shantytowns they dubbed "Hoovervilles" in gratitude to the man they held responsible. Wink.

Al Capone himself probably helped more unhoused poor in the Chicago soup kitchen he started than Hoover did in his presidency.

In 1963, Kennedy passed the Community Health Act, which he deemed a remarkable success. The Act ushered former institutionalized patients to community-based homes; these received funding but nowhere near enough. Many of the affected in larger cities ended up on the streets, for without community support, the mentally ill have more trouble getting treatment, maintaining medication regimens, and supporting themselves.

Such information reveals a lot about our communities and the motivations of their inhabitants. A reevaluation of our priorities, more attention to our inner gardens and the communities surrounding them, and a dash of kindness could go a long way if we choose to let it – just a thought.

Homelessness reached new plateaus in the 1980s, thanks to President Reagan. Cuts on housing and social services resulted in a deficit of 3.3 million domiciles. The resulting increase in the unsheltered still managed to surprise many.

By now, it should be clear that none of these facts add up to support the common assumption that the unhoused are outside because they want to be.

My wife and I were never homeless in the conventional sense, but the truth touched us as if we, in fact, did live on the street. We both recognized that governments cared little for average Joes and Janes and, moreover, both of us always felt like aliens growing up: as if we were on the outside looking in.

In addition, many times we found ourselves in Asia, America, or elsewhere and wondered how we should afford a flight/bus ride out or even the next meal. This understanding gave us the experience to say that one reason why people rove the streets is because house-dwellers *need* someone to be out there.

No matter how horrible life is in our home, they think we're still better off than The Unfortunates out in the cold.

In the 1990s, new homeless shelters and soup kitchens popped up across the country, but providing emergency services did little to stem the flow of down-and-outers: numbers of unsheltered persons still rose and remained high. It was apparent these people needed more than "soap, soup, and salvation"– the Salvation Army's recipe for the solution.

Like many other problems in this world – medical conditions, national conflicts, etc. – our governments' proposed solutions often amounted to Band-Aids, and to an empty, "Take two aspirins and call me in the morning." Dealing with symptoms is so much easier than addressing causes.

Meanwhile, guys like Luke (not his real name), all of twenty-one, are left to ask us one night at the edge of Germany's Black Forest if we could spare some change for a meal; the park in front of the Sacred Heart of Jesus Church in nearby Freiburg was overrun by young men afraid to look us in the eye; almost every underpass and bridge in San Francisco is decorated with ragged tents and shopping carts; the train stations of the world are backdrops for another heroin user to run across; the children in Cairo, Marrakesh, and Port au Prince follow tourists with hope in their eyes and air in their bellies.

I recall an older gentleman asking us for change in Oakland. After informing him we had none, he answered, "But I'm homeless."

"Technically, we are too," I answered.

That man could have turned angrily and maybe cursed us, but instead, he wished us a great day and went on his wandering way.

In the 1980s, cuts to federal low-income housing programs drove homelessness to new heights; in this young century, the housing crisis – i.e., greed – fuels another rise. Delegates named "Lack of available and affordable housing" a major cause of vagrancy at the 2004 United States Conference of Mayors. No one wanted low-income housing in upscale residential areas, while in other places, the biggest names on Wall Street purchased an unprecedented amount of real estate. Such firms, sadly, hardly symbolize generosity.

For example, it is common business practice for landlords in poverty-stricken communities to raise rent as a counterbalance to "risky investments." Lo and behold, more profits are reaped from cheaper housing than properties in more affluent areas. Experts claim such deplorable behavior "results in…hardship and is a source of residential insecurity, eviction, and homelessness."

Other causes for this problem exist, but feel free to peruse the list[22]. Precious few unhoused people are in the street because they choose to be. At the top of the food chain, politicians on both sides debate endlessly and accomplish little. Worse, our competitive, materialistic culture keeps apathy and a lack of pity common denominators in

---

[22] https://en.wikipedia.org/wiki/Homelessness_in_the_United_States#Causes.

many of our lives and divides communities with an ever-present self-centered mentality.

The housed are too tired, busy, and uninformed to care about the 582,462 people on American streets every night[23], while the unhoused remain disturbed and ill, without roofs, plumbing, heating, healthy food options, and the means to avoid their fates.

We sought to escape these harsh truths by leaving in the first place. After traveling so many miles and visiting so many places, we found the effects of greed waited for us patiently everywhere.

Jack Everly ~ *I thank my wife and daughters for making our adventures something truly special.*

---

[23] In January 2022, for example.

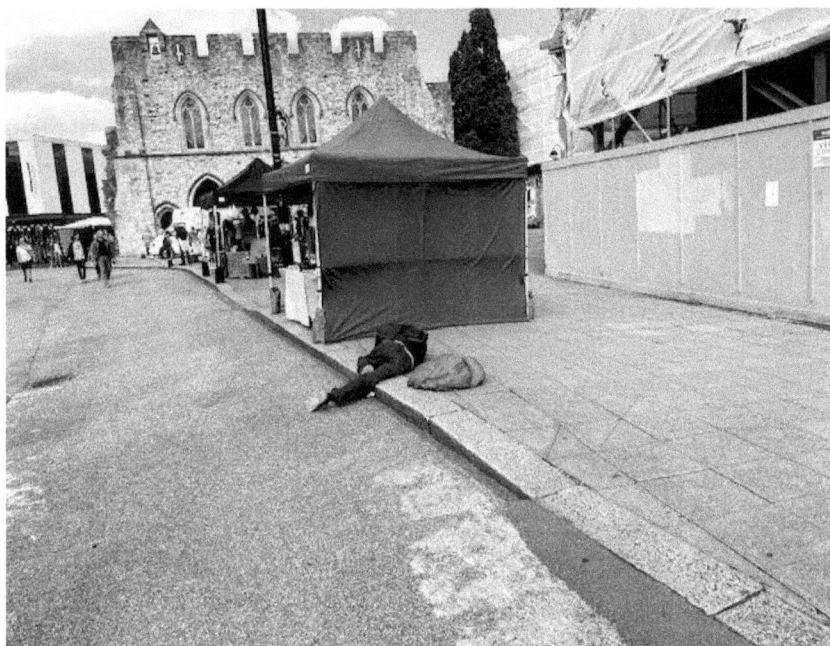

United Kingdom
Dennis Pitocco, Photographer

The Blue Man

By Karin vonKrenner
Southwest France

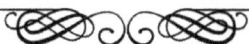

❦

In every grain of sand, lies the memory of mountains.

Karin vonKrenner

*I*n the bustling heart of this old city, history is etched deep into every cracked cathedral stone and cobbled step. The dark past is lit now by the delighted awe of selfie-clicking tourists. Festooned market stalls laden with flowers and heart-shaped pretzels circle the square, and music mixes across the river from overflowing cafes. An endless dance of waiters carrying tiered ice cream and cake seems to dish out joy with every sweet spoonful.

In the recess of a shop corner untouched by the sun, sits a man. He is a shadow of silence, a world unto himself.

He is ragdoll still, disconnected
from the life flowing past him.

A man of enigmatic presence, dressed in faded fabrics that once bore the vibrancy of a different life. His beard, tangled and long, has become a testament to time's passage. It frames a countenance marked by the weight of a journey that transcended borders. A face folded into a dirt-encrusted map of his own unwritten history. Tired shoulders slump into the wall, seeking harsh comfort in cold stone.

Within the twists of his greying hair, strands of stories are woven, whispering of lands traversed, and hopes once cradled close to the heart. Heavy eyebrows, furrowed by the burden of an uncertain fate, frame eyes that hold the wisdom of silence and the sorrow of forgotten dreams.

It is his eyes that resonate with the essence of his existence. An ethereal depth that could crack the very soul of the world.

In the dim, cold corner, he is almost invisible, just a low outline against the blue wall. Detached, disconnected from the bright world swirling beyond the shadows. So small a distance to create such an impenetrable distance between worlds. The golden festooned doors of the prestigious Galeria department store spill sparkling light onto snowy streets. But not on him. The chills of this foreign winter creep and claw at his weary bones, a bitter reminder of estrangement from warmth and family.

In my approach, his eyes flicker alive with fear.

I have acknowledged his presence beyond the tossing of coins. I see him. I can feel his sudden, strong sense of heightened wariness as I crouch down before him. My skin tingles from my own caution as if approaching a feral city cat. Instinctually, we assess each other as potential threats before habituating into accepted behavior patterns. Violence is not the social norm here, only apathy.

His face mesmerizes me, so many stories flickering behind the mask of indifference. Reaching into my backpack, I slowly pull out my camera showing it to him. For the first time, he looks straight at me. In that look is a returned acknowledgment, a spark of life. Now, we see each other. An exchange, as old as human history can record. Take and give.

His hand stretches out for money. In return for a story and photos, I accept, and the flash of my camera draws him into a focus of light, briefly reclaiming him from the shadows.

His body shrinks into his coat ever so slightly with a deep sigh, as if the effort of speaking deflates him. His name has been lost in the shadows of his journey here, abandoned and forgotten by the years away from home and a distance too far to ever return. The polished colors of his memories have been deleted; only greyed shades remain, and the truth of them is no longer certain. That man in those memories has gone forever.

He tells a story of hope crushed by a crueler fate.

A story and words recited around the world in every language. He ventured across borders from a small, warm Italian village, searching for new work to frame a better life. Yet, this country was not kind to him, finding no value in his skills or life. Barred by language and culture, doors did not open. They closed.

The promises of work and prosperity whispered in his ears dissolved soon after his arrival, leaving him stranded without money and diminishing hopes, pushing him daily, weekly, and monthly toward the harsh world of homelessness and begging.

When dawn breaks in his corner, he watches the city come alive, a silent spectator to the flurry of other incomprehensible worlds bustling past him. Every day, he marks the untouchable opulence flowing through the grand store doors, a parade of people who carefully avoid glancing toward his weathered figure. He knows them all, the hassled employees rushing to and from the trains. The patrons move rigidly as if power is a heavy weight pulling at their feet. He is a ghost among the living as if the invisible force of homelessness blocks him from the gaze of all who walk past. He sees them all, unseen.

His heart aches not just for the warmth of shelter but for the fading memories of his distant family. Once, he was loved. With every passing hour and day, the wall of silence separates him further from his past and any who knew him—crushing him deeper into the ground. Perhaps, now, they have resigned themselves to the idea of his demise. Death by absence. Better they fill their voids of grief and uncertainty with an idea of death—his gift to them.

The richly dressed businessmen with glittering wives glide by, enveloped in bubbles of privilege, eyes fixed on the sparkling window displays and the allure of luxuries within. The chatter of parties and holidays stream past him. A slight quickening of footsteps was their only acknowledgment of his ephemeral existence.

In the retreat of his corner, there are brief moments of solace. Amidst the pitiless alienation, there are moments of fleeting human connection. An awkward nod from a passer-by tossing change at his feet. A child pulling toward him despite a parent dragging them off as if poverty is an untouchable disease. Fractional moments in endless days to bridge the vast expanse between his world and theirs. So close, so far. Light to dark.

He doesn't belong in this foreign country and has been forgotten and discarded by its exclusive society, labeled with resentment as "Auslander," outsider. Yet, in the depths of his being, he still grasps a flickering hope of being seen, acknowledged, and perhaps embraced. A day where he is not an obstacle on the pavement but a human yearning to belong once more.

A reason not to die.

He waves me away, exhausted by the effort of remembering shredded memories. I empty the rest of my pocket money into his plastic cup. It will change nothing in either of our lives. I will still carry a burden of guilt for what I cannot do. He will be cold and hungry again tomorrow. Turning away toward my own precarious life. I only know one thing: "There, but for the grace of God, go I."

Every day, I pass by, and he remains in the same corner. I leave a hot coffee by his side and continue on my own way. He does not acknowledge me again and remains the silent guardian of his own story, waiting amidst the symphony of hurried footsteps for something we fail to give him.

One day, he was gone. I don't know what happened to him; nobody could even recall his existence. All that is left is a story and a photograph—an epitaph in memory of the Blue Man.

Man in the street. Still unknown.

Emerging from the Dark: Re-entry into Society

By Zeina Navia
Canada

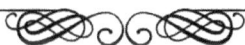

I am a divine being meant to serve, guide, and mentor others.

Zeina Navia

I ended up unhoused/homeless in the summer of 2022 for 12 weeks. I started over, leaving everything behind except a knapsack and one bag. While hiking, I lost my wallet and ID, forcing me to hitchhike to where I live now.

Work was not easy to obtain, although tons of jobs were out there, supposedly. I applied to close to 150. In order to have some money for things not provided for by local services and resources, I took a lawn-care job part-time. While being unhoused, I made tons of friends and really learned what homelessness/being unhoused was about. *Only by living the reality can one truly understand it.*

People judge, have misconceptions, label all homeless as druggies who just want things for free and are troublesome. I have heard people describe a sense of entitlement and too much access to things. These are NOT true and NOT reality. Many were like me and ended up homeless because of illness, loss of a job, relocation, ending of a marriage or romantic relationship, dabbling in drugs, gambling, or alcohol, and then did not know how to get out of it.

Like all of us, many unhoused have low moments, negative thoughts running through their heads, lack self-worth, and have lost faith in themselves, the system, and society. I have seen individuals walk by a homeless person on the street, say they do not have cash to give, etc. I understand the hesitation about giving cash as you do not know where it goes, but how about buying a homeless person a meal, a cup of coffee, or sharing a food resource?

Unhoused Time

Homelessness was not as bad as I thought it might be, but again, for me, it was summer. I come from a helping/ customer service background, so I asked questions, looked into resources, met with professionals, and questioned if something did not make sense to me. I located food, clothing, shelter resources, places where one could get water, a shower, part-time work, and charity to assist one along their journey.

Affordable housing does not exist unless you literally turn yourself and your life over to the government. It means endless paperwork, meetings with government workers or local social service staff, and being put on a waitlist for months or years for low-cost or transitional housing. If you have lots of money, you can rent easily. The other solution is to live with roommates.

I borrowed some money or assisted those with disabilities to earn some money for things I could not get from a shelter or charity. As I lost my ID, I could not access my banking account until a new photo ID was obtained. My cell phone was stolen. I went without a phone for a few weeks until I had earned enough money to buy an inexpensive one. I went to the library, the local work organization to check my email, and Starbucks to use WIFI.

I looked for housing and contacted a few friends so they knew I was alive and had relocated. This process to obtain a new ID took almost six months for some reason. Supposedly, a new license was mailed to the shelter where I stayed but never arrived. I just went and ordered yet another. Three months later, it showed up.

I located all the thrift shops in the city, came across a local used-book store, and many small local shops, and met such warm and caring souls. My world shifted, and in the end, it all worked out for me. BUT it was not handed to me on a silver platter. I worked for it. While it was suggested numerous times that I go on Welfare or Disability for a steady income, I refused. While I have health challenges, I am not disabled, nor do I see myself that way. Mindset is a choice.

Many suggested I have a "sugar daddy," and again, I refused. I would take care of myself and reach out to resources as needed. I do not just turn to the government or a man to provide for me. I was not raised this way. Plus, my marriages proved to me that I could not rely on men. When the going got tough, they disappeared emotionally, physically, and financially; they used me, abused me, and left me in financial ruin. Me, I just kept plugging along. My spirit is strong.

Men solicited me and wanted to pursue a physical relationship. I was not seeking this, and I am not a casual gal. I made sure all of the unhoused knew I did not do drugs, never tried them, and did not smoke weed or cigarettes. Yes, I liked a beer or a shot of whiskey sometimes… but I valued myself enough not to sell myself or my integrity.

Now, I am thriving, and I did it because I pushed myself and reached out to the agencies and resources that understood. I advocated for something that was lacking or did not make sense. I asked questions. I did not accept the protocol or path a homeless person was "supposed" to take, as suggested to me by a few. I used my voice to obtain what was needed and to share what was unfair and unjust.

A friend who protected me when I was homeless died this past winter out in the cold. It should not have happened. Shelters closed their doors to him because he had some issues. The last time I saw him, he was lucid, clean, and wanting to change his life. The church I am a member of runs a hot meal program every Sunday, and this is the last place I saw him. Again, on that day, at that moment, he was lucid and clean.

I painted a painting in his memory and donated it to my church. I wanted to capture his essence and caring vibes/attitude. We need more people like this who just care with no strings attached.

Everyone deserves access to the basics regardless of their socioeconomic situation.

The "Tree of Life" to me has many meanings, but one of them that I interpret is "As above, so below," meaning that no matter how rich or poor, we all deserve a safe and affordable home, clothing, food, education, and transportation – the basics. Add in care, compassion, understanding, love, friendship, and health; we are all wealthy.

Shelters are not all they are made out to be, and they are all different. Sleeping in a room with 15-20 other people is not easy, especially when you are the only female. I was grateful for the roof over my head, the relatively comfortable mat, the air conditioning in summer, food, clothing, companionship, activities, and some helpful staff.

One wonders why some staff work there, though, as their hearts were not in it. To them, it is a paycheck; to me, that is the wrong attitude. Find employment that brings you joy and happiness. If being a janitor fills your soul, do that job. If dealing with numbers all day lights up your soul, do that job.

A staff member banned me from the shelter for 24 hours as I stood up for an older, unhoused soul who did something nice. He and I slept in the park that night. I went back the next day to get on the waitlist and, through the speaker (not face to face), was told by another staff member that I was banned for a week without explanation.

I chose the streets and parks as I require solitude, peace, quiet, and my own schedule. The shelters had childish curfews – in by 9 PM, and one must be up by 6:30 AM. We are adults and should be treated as such. The world desires control. Time schedules should be flexible, understanding, and compassionate.

When I was homeless/unhoused, I had three friends who offered money with no strings attached, to which I said no but thanked them.

I had another who insisted I stay in a hotel room for one night toward the end of my homelessness so I could sleep in a proper bed, take a hot shower, meditate, and enjoy solitude in the air conditioning. After being offered five times, I finally accepted.

One of my friends recently asked me a question: "Why did you not accept the money? The universe was putting people in your path to help you." I thought about it and told him I could not accept the money as I did not believe it was part of the divine plan for me. I had food, shelter (although it happened to be outside), clothing, friends, a place to cool off (library or mall), and a part-time job – the basics. I was enjoying nature, the warm weather, and freedom. Overall, I was happy during this time. I thought of myself as camping. Besides working 16 hours a week, my time was mine to do as I wanted.

My last three nights being unhoused were the toughest of the twelve weeks. I was exhausted at this point and fell asleep out in the open but in a safe space. I remember waking up after a few hours and seeing a few younger guys sitting on bikes nearby. When I sat up, they asked me if I was okay. I remember saying I was exhausted and went back to sleep.

They kept watching over me.

The next night, I slept on a set of cement steps with my belongings close by. On my final night, I stayed on a park bench where I knew I would be safe as it was outside a church. I hardly slept and was physically, emotionally, and spiritually exhausted. At some point during the night, the sprinklers came on, and my stuff and I got wet, and I could not have cared less.

A friend contacted me that night, and we texted back and forth. He wanted me off the streets and was trying to build up my inner reserve about finding employment. (I had been working a part-time seasonal job that ended suddenly.) I was busy applying for other jobs and waiting for one to appear.

It was cold these three nights as the weather was turning. It was September. I attempted to get into a local shelter a few times, putting my pride aside, but I was told it was full. I found out later this was not the case. So again, two local shelters provided services but chose to let me sleep outside, both knowing my health issues and why I was unhoused. I told them both I would never set foot inside or request their services again.

At the end of my three months, I was couch surfing for a few weeks until I found my current lodgings. I am grateful to those two people who offered me a couch to sleep on. Many others knew of my circumstances and never once offered me their couch or space on their living room floor. They would text me to see how I was managing in the cooler weather and ask if I was okay.

I was initially disappointed and then realized I was judging, which was not okay. They had their reasons. As I live by the "treat others as you want to be treated" rule, I would have opened my home to a friend in two seconds with rules, boundaries, and expectations. Others do not live by this rule, though. It is what it is.

We all have a unique path. We all have choices, but I am at peace with my decisions. I forgive myself for any choices or decisions I made. I forgive all those who hurt me in the past – left me, abused me, and were not there for me when I was ill, sick, or unhoused.

I will be the light that shines for others and guide them on a healing path if they choose this option. I have faith. I know all will be okay and work out, and I will continue to follow my dreams, intuition, and inner guidance. I plant seeds for others, let them ruminate, and think about what I have said. Perhaps they will come across a different result, and that is okay.

I made and still make it a point to check in with those who are homeless (unhoused) and let them know there are resources. I guide them, listen to them, and just hold space for them. I do not judge them if they use drugs or alcohol. I share concerns if they go overboard, though, which just means I care.

**There is a camaraderie between
the homeless or the unhoused.**

One checks in on others, ensures they have food, clothing, a place to get clean, and offers support. Sometimes, $3 or $5 is given so someone can get a hot coffee or something small to eat, or I will bring food to someone or take them in to get breakfast or lunch.

Be a light shining in the darkness and shine brighter. Never stop loving or caring for one another. Open your homes to each other and share your food. Each of us has been given a gift. Use it to serve one another.

Zeina Navia ~ *I thank divine-the creator, local people who helped me, and friends who offered assistance near and far*

Descendants of the Unsheltered

By Sha'Kiera Star
Texas, USA

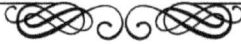

A wise girl knows her limits.
A smart girl knows she has none.

Marilyn Monroe

We are the most vulnerable of society
Children with eyes that see poverty with promise
Pure at heart, we love Mom and Dad no matter what

We eat scraps gracefully and with glee
Go without for parents in need
Take on a paternal role to siblings

There are times when we are 2nd to the drugs
3rd to the man, 4th to unemployment, we try to understand
Sit silently in the shadow while you're asking for a hand
And we know we'll never be 1ˢᵗ

We were the future, but what kind of future is to come
We slum in the ghetto nest that breeds greed and hopelessness

We dream sweet dreams but can't profess
The night covers and shields us
We rest in the hands of the creator

Now I lay me down to sleep
I pray the Lord I'm safe at peace
Whatever I need, when I rise
May God see me through and be close by my side

What doesn't break you shakes you.

"I pacify the damage that haunts me with the intensity of my voice and a vengeance toward my past."

When we are born, I do not believe that we are automatically prone to fear, equipped with faith, or guided by hope. I also contend that innocence shields some of the harshness that reality will surely bring our way. My upbringing catapulted me into being exposed to drugs, violence, and instability. I say that today with an appreciation for that truth.

I was never shielded from the cruelty of the world but fueled by one's disparity, which holds a special place in my story. I am the daughter of unfulfilled talent and stolen time. My mother had this mantra: "Never forget where you come from." With every jarring life lesson, I thought that her advice was counterproductive to who I would become as a woman.

On the contrary, there is internal power for anyone who makes it out of trying circumstances beyond their control. In my case, I experienced various situations where my parents were either absent or impaired and unable to provide suitable living conditions or nourishment. In hindsight, I share my testimony, unashamed about where I come from. I may not be unscathed from trauma; however, I am empowered to appreciate the trajectory of my life. Being inadequately sheltered was cold, removed the possibility of a healthy environment, and increased the odds of failure.

Through therapy, I was told that I have harbored and carried the younger me within throughout the years. She is protected by each version of me that I become. I have promised her an abundant life. I pacify the damage that haunts her with the intensity of my voice and a vengeance toward my past.

I am thankful for lights when I click a switch, and I can appreciate candles when there is no electricity. Covers and warmth from a thermostat shield me from the cold, but I have kept warm from heat from a blow dryer. If I say so myself, I've become a next-level home cook and enjoy trying new recipes. I have also stood in line for free food and made do with just enough or none at all. When I rest at night, I am grateful for clean linens, pillows, and a real mattress. I have also slept on my share of floors with my head propped against my arm as a makeshift pillow.

I have honored my mother's lesson. I have not forgotten where I come from. I embrace it! What doesn't break you shapes you, and that's a fact.

The Wonder Years

I wiped my mom's tears at night, and my mom wiped mine. We bonded through our pain and displacement, silently with more suffering to come over time.

The terror invaded my small body as I stepped down from the back step. I walked cautiously, holding my younger brother's hand. I heard the arguing from the bedroom window, but it wasn't until the screams began that my curiosity caused me to pursue the noise coming from out back. The image of my mother in distress triggered instincts that were unfamiliar to me as a child.

My eyes quickly scanned the backyard. I tried to process the rage that I was witnessing. I vaguely recall spectators, but no one intervened. Today, cell phones would have recorded the beating, this page of my life. Instead, I have a photographic memory of this tragedy.

That wasn't the first time that I saw my mom being assaulted, and it wouldn't be the finale. She noticed us at some point in the fighting. I'm sure my brother's cry and my screaming for her broke the sound barrier that only a mother could penetrate. She flailed her arms at the man and fought back fiercely to no avail. With what must have been her protective impulse and with us in harm's way, she signaled for me to run toward my grandfather's old Ford F-150 parked nearby.

I followed instructions, running as quickly as my legs would carry me. I could taste the salt from the tears that made their way to my lips. My mother somehow escaped the fury of fists, punches, and slaps that brutalized her small frame in just enough time to lock herself inside of the truck as well. Her nickname was Rock, short for Raquel and symbolic of her life. I felt the name was fitting and, by my definition, means "to endure emotional or physical pain without perishing." We were all panicking, but there was some relief when she made her way inside the truck's cab.

I gripped her torso like I was trying to re-enter her body, a safe space. She assured me with a lie that we would be ok; I had no choice but to believe her as evidence that she was still breathing, still fighting, still by our side. She removed her shirt, barely able to raise her arms above her head.

She started to wrap her left wrist with the fabric using her dominant right hand. That's when I noticed that she was injured and had a gaping cut on her wrist. She said, "Help Mommy and pull this tight." I pulled the red cloth that was once white with all of my might. I touched her back, and blood oozed, warming my hands like sand.

The rest is cloudy, but when I heard the sirens, I welcomed the cavalry. The paramedics worked on her immediately, and finally, I exhaled. When I recalled this incident, I called my uncle in tears. There was no answer. He was the man who beat my mother that day. I don't know what I would have said; we have yet to have that discussion. The dysfunction in my family is so deep that as the years went on, it was as if it never happened, which perpetuated the fact that it continued.

The hospital arranged for us to go to a shelter. The next day, we entered the doors of a large building that reminded me of a warehouse. A kind woman who managed the facility checked us in. My mom was so weak. I helped wherever possible, mostly being an authoritative figure for my brother or an extra set of hands when I saw her struggle. We were escorted to a large room filled with women and children in double digits.

I wondered if what happened to us happened to them. I didn't understand the magnitude of our homelessness. I would like to distinguish that there are levels to being unsheltered. As a reminder, today, I can feel the discomfort and sadness that flood my memory when I see mothers alongside their children holding up signs at a busy intersection. It's the same feeling I've carried since the day we entered the shelter.

We were assigned one cot for the three of us. I lay back to my mother's chest, and my brother's back to mine. It was the closest we'd ever been, and I cherish that memory. I wiped my mom's tears at night, and my mom wiped mine. We bonded through our pain and displacement, silently with more suffering to come over time.

We continued a course of intermittent housing and unsheltered moments throughout my upbringing. We lived a bit of a transient lifestyle as my mother tried to make a life in Texas, Illinois, and New York.

Stars don't shine without darkness.

"I felt inadequate, and I did not believe that I could be any more than I was — NO ONE."

My teenage years were a passage of some sort. I survived a vulnerable stage intact. I understood from my surroundings that I desired more. My spirit survived what my heart could not. Somehow, my tenacity would surpass my grief.

My father was serving a 10-year sentence in Jackson State Penitentiary for armed robbery, and my mother had succumbed to her drug addiction. This left my brother and me in the care of family at times. That in itself was an unsheltered reality. If there is no place like home, there is no feeling like not having one. I remember several months without my mom and having been placed with my great-grandmother.

There must have been about 10 of us living in her modest home. I overheard my aunt say that my mom was locked away in a mental hospital. I didn't understand. I loathed being estranged from my mother. Later, I learned that the claim was true. She never gained resources to address her mental health issues. Growing up, I knew we were poor; we lived an uprooted lifestyle. Through it all, I also knew that she loved me. It is the one unconditional sentiment that I miss about her.

Still, I can admit I resented the impact that her lifestyle had on mine. I became masterful at avoiding my mother when she was high. This left me to my own adolescent devices and neighborhood influences. I hung out with the local gang and learned survival tactics as I acquainted myself with the streets. Ironically, exposure to crime, barely escaping sexual assault, and being jumped by six girls would be an effective lesson for me. Wrong crowd, wrong time, attending school periodically, I was lost.

My grades suffered immensely, and there was no consequence or acknowledgment of my lack of engagement from any adult close in proximity. At this time, my grandmother rented the home where we resided. We were years away from the time spent in the shelter, yet our outlook was bleak. I underperformed throughout my high school career, drinking to numb my pain. I was becoming no one. I felt inadequate, and I did not believe that I could be any more than I was.

I vividly remember being so hungry during class that I could not concentrate. By this time, my mother was a diagnosed alcoholic and suffered from pancreatitis, which led to her being hospitalized frequently. This, on top of the continued drug abuse and manic episodes, made it difficult to balance her good days when she was sober, read us stories from her journal, or cook dinner.

I left my mother's house when I was 16 years old. She lashed out at me that day. I remember how hard I hit the stairs while running away from her. Emotionally, the toll was too heavy. Physically, I'd had enough. I endured being the target of her anger for too long. But in reality, that made me stronger. I took a stance for the first time — a prelude into adulthood.

I chose to wander and not be still. I found different places to dwell. My best friend Crea was caring enough to convince her mother to let me stay over many nights. She never asked why. I think she saw the trouble in my eyes and pitied me. I was a polite kid, very tolerable.

I jumped couches for a while with one promise I'd made myself. I refused to go back to my mom's house. In my senior year, I attracted the attention of a man 15 years older than me. I had minimal contact with my family, which made it easy to manipulate me. He was educated, studious, and exciting. I secretly stayed at his home and accepted the facade of being cared for and loved. As a young woman, I subconsciously felt drawn to what I saw as fatherlike love. Of course, I was wrong.

Soon after we were acquainted, he revealed to me that he smoked crack cocaine. This was after I was groomed and promised a future together. When he pulled out his pipe in front of me and lit it, I became nauseous and small.

The smell of crack was familiar to my sense of smell. I was eight years old again, looking at my mama high and free in her own way. I stood across from him as his brain floated, and he sank into the couch. Mouth open, eyes wide shut, it sickened me. I found myself walking the streets at 2:00 a.m. aimlessly, car after car pulling up to me and driving away after realizing I wasn't a prostitute. I was alone and unsheltered.

Becoming Me

No food, no bed, no money, no chance. The shelter, overcrowded spaces, floors of family members, and couches of friends and foes were "enough" for me. I emerged from walking the streets scared and out of place with a plan, a vision. I refused the path of the inner city. Young people in my neighborhood died frequently. I wanted to live. I still do!

I went on to earn my high school diploma and entered the workforce on a mission. I learned the business world by entering professional spaces that seemed to be for those who profited from people like me. I learned from the inside out. I learned quickly that my leadership was innate. It was evident in how others took to me.

I became what I call a "Corporate Grad." I progressed through a series of jobs, gained leadership experience, and have discovered a career as a life coach, an award-winning trainer, and a certified Diversity, Equity, and Inclusion professional.

The greatest treasure through this entire hardship was finding my voice. I tackled open mic venues around Detroit and discovered expressions far beyond my journal and the short stories, raps, and poems I secretly wrote. That was the beginning of my healing. Supporting myself was a welcomed challenge and encouraged me to continue. I stumbled often, but I also discovered people who believed I could be more significant than my past.

During the past year, I launched a public speaking career. It embraces both my spoken-word origins and corporate acuity. I use my hard-earned wisdom and street-smart sense of humor to highlight blind spots, misaligned business structures, and lingering social biases.

I may be a descendant of the unsheltered. But I've sheltered myself and my son as an adult. And I am a vessel to help others find refuge and a better path forward.

Homeless in the Dunes

By Matt Love
Southern Oregon Coast, USA

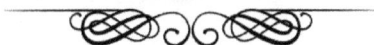

"So you know where the official homeless camps are in town?" said a woman's voice at the counter of an animal welfare thrift store in Gold Beach.

It was a dry and balmy Saturday, an October afternoon, in a town of fewer than 2000 on the remote southern Oregon coast, and I was browsing the store's selection of VHS tapes.

Did Gold Beach have official sites for homeless people to camp? Impossible. A town this size?

I heard the clerk describe three such places.

Three?! Portland doesn't have even one. In this extremely conservative beach town in the extremely conservative Curry County? No way.

I eased around a corner to better eavesdrop. I heard "near the hospital," "Fifth Street," and "airport," and that was it. I then noticed the woman asking about the camps and the man beside her. They were Gold Beach residents or used to be. I recognized them from various local dive bars during my multiple stays in Gold Beach over the recent years. He was a Grateful Dead fanatic, and she worked as a waitress at the most expensive restaurant in town. Both were in their 50s.

**They now exuded the unmistakable
vibe of being homeless.**

I left the store and walked to my vehicle. Parked next to mine was a red sedan I knew belonged to the couple of years ago. I inspected it. Sure enough, they were living out of it and most likely were returning to town and looking for a place to crash.

What had happened to them?

I drove away and to the bookstore. A good friend manages it, and I knew she would give me the lowdown on these official campsites in Gold Beach.

She did, somewhat, but there was confusion. Were there three or five, or were they even up and running at all? She also told me a rumor flying around town that some homeless advocate from Gold Beach was driving to Portland and transporting homeless people to Gold Beach because there was money in it from the state.

Total bullshit, of course. I hear this in every rural Oregon town I visit. They just can't admit it's their own people suffering, and they almost always are from the town where they ended up homeless. The rural politicians and social media pundits love to blame Blue Portland and liberals for the homelessness in their own Red communities. It's so easy that way.

I drove around the hospital and didn't see anything that looked like a sanctioned site for the homeless to camp. There were no tents anywhere. I did see, however, two or three vehicles that were clearly being used as domiciles.

Next, I drove toward Fifth Street, which looked like a dead end from Highway 101. It was near the high school, the public works department, and a sewage treatment plant. The airport was around there, too, but I didn't see anything, so I turned around in the parking lot of a grocery store and drove to check in to my motel. I was exhausted after six hours of driving.

I checked in, ate a snack, and tried watching some football, but I felt restless as dusk approached. There was a story about Oregon's homeless nearby, and I wanted to find it.

Shoe leather time. I donned my pea coat and headed on foot to the hospital. It's the only way to investigate a story. So there I was, on foot, seeking a story about homelessness. I was supposed to be there for recreation and relaxation and not thinking about, interacting with, or writing about the crisis.

Fat chance. It's everywhere in Oregon.

I walked around the hospital and down a few side roads that narrowed into housing, the willows, and the woods. Nothing.

An older man in uniform stood out behind the hospital, dumping garbage into a dumpster. I approached him and saw his ID badge that read "Housekeeper."

I introduced myself as a writer working on a book about the homeless in Oregon. Did he know anything about the alleged sanctioned homeless encampments in the area?

Yeah, he knew a lot about homelessness in Gold Beach. It was all around him and part of the hospital's day-to-day operation. We talked for 20 minutes as the light faded. This is what he told me:

> Sometimes, the church next door lets homeless people camp or park their cars on its property. But they have to leave every morning and can't leave anything behind. Maybe that's one of the official sites? Check the dunes near the south end of the airport. I haven't seen it, but that's what I've heard. We have homeless people coming to the emergency room all the time. Usually, the same people. They show up, or the cops and EMTs bring them.

> We do what we can and then discharge them after a few days. A couple died not too long ago, right after being discharged. Their bodies were found in the bushes down by the river. Exposure. We don't have anyone on staff like a social worker to find them housing. There is no housing. I think someone is doing something in the City, but I don't know anything about that.

I thanked him for the information. It was too dark to visit the airport, so I returned to the motel.

In the morning, while carrying a cup of coffee, I walked to the airport searching for the homeless encampment.

I found it.

Fifth Street was dead-ended at the beach. A barricade blocked vehicles from driving on the sand. Someone had spray-painted ALOHA on the barricade.

The encampment amounted to five tents pitched at angles in the dunes. It had a million-dollar view of the ocean, and it was rolling white, slate, and loud on a dry and bright morning when I stood in front of the site. The airport runway was to my back. The high school football field was a hundred yards away.

I saw the remains of a few campfires. Garbage was strewn about. There were no dumpsters or portable toilets. No water. No power. No pallets to pitch tents on.

This place was an official site. I surmised the City simply made this piece of public property available, understanding that the cops wouldn't hassle the residents and they wouldn't be squatting on private property. But the City apparently wasn't going to provide anything more because, as the conventional wisdom goes, that enables and attracts more homeless people. I really don't know if that is true or not. I do know if you don't provide a few basic necessities, there is still homelessness, and its squalor is intensified.

No one was stirring in the encampment. I felt a little strange doing so, but I took out my phone and snapped a few photographs.

I wanted to talk to someone, but it's not like you can go up and knock on someone's tent and introduce yourself as a writer about Oregon's homelessness crisis. Sure, I could have done exactly that, but I didn't. I wasn't feeling it. I want my interactions to be spontaneous and not an editorial errand.

What would these residents do when they awakened? Two inches of rain was forecast for the evening. Do homeless people take walks on

Oregon's public ocean beaches? Sure they do. I've seen it for years. They collect agates and limpets, and party in driftwood forts. They run their dogs and play ball and stick with them. They also fish for perch and crab off docks and jetties.

I didn't stay long. True, it wasn't much of site, but the Pacific was right there as a neighbor and perhaps a counselor. It seemed much better to me than living under an off-ramp to an Interstate Highway in Portland.

A half hour later, I was walking through the dunes of another beach, Bailey Beach, across the Rogue River. I was killing time before a coffee date with a good friend.

I saw a vehicle parked in the dunes, 20 feet from the beach, and approached it: a Ford Bronco 2000, battered, rusted, duct-taped, bald tires, Washington plates, expired tags. A mobile domicile for sure. They all have that look.

Nothing stirred around it. I peered inside the driver-side window. The passenger seat was crammed with stuff.

I hit the beach and saw a man playing stick with a dog and assumed they were the inhabitants of the Bronco.

After a 15-minute walk, I returned to my car via a path through the dunes. The Bronco was blocking the way, but I kept heading in that direction. The man materialized with his dog. His back was to me. The dog was a pit bull mix and wore a coat. The dog saw me and bolted my way. He didn't seem angry, and I greeted him like an old friend.

The man called out to the dog. I met the dog, and he was an old softy. Then, I met the man near his rig and a woman in the back seat. She called out a hello from a half-open back door, and I caught a glimpse of her wrapped in a blanket.

They were in their 30s/40s and evinced a post-meth look. His cheeks were sallow. Her face was riddled with scars. They didn't seem high at all. They looked totally exhausted.

I asked how it was going. I said I couldn't imagine how they survived. They said it was hard. I got their story, at least part of it:

The couple had been homeless for about a year and were from the general area. They were broken, and the Bronco had run out of gas. Tomorrow, they had an appointment to meet some homeless advocate in Gold Beach who might be able to help them find housing. Was there such housing in Gold Beach? They didn't know.

I asked if they got into housing, were they going to look for work. I don't know why I asked that—it just popped out because I had seen *Help Wanted* signs all over Gold Beach. They kind of nodded to that question. I didn't press. There was no way they could live out of the Bronco and work a minimum-wage job. They needed somewhere to clean up, rally, and get their bearings.

"My heart breaks for you and others," I said. It felt weird and corny saying that, but it's what came out.

"It's tough," the man said.

I fished out seven bucks and handed it over to the man.

"Thank you," he said. The woman thanked me, too.

Then I dug out a $20 and gave it to him. "Get some gas and make the appointment," I said. "Get something for the dog, too."

The man thanked me again. We shook hands. I wished them good luck. I returned the next morning, intending to give them some power bars and dog food. They were gone.

Nowhere to Call Home

Living with the insecurity, anxiety, and possibility of becoming unsheltered

By Noreen Braman
Brooklyn, Middlesex NY, New Jersey, USA

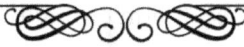

To save a life is a real and beautiful thing. To make a home
for the homeless, yes, it is a thing that must be good;
whatever the world may say, it cannot be wrong.

~ Vincent Van Gogh

"You either shape up or ship out!" These words were not being shouted at some unfortunate Marine Corps recruit. My stepfather aimed them at 11-year-old me. "We could just leave you here," he yelled. The threat was terrifying. Would I wake up one morning to find everyone gone, leaving me to fend for myself? Would I become the Crazy Old Baby Carriage Lady?

We were kids who didn't understand or know better. Crazy Old Baby Carriage Lady regularly appeared in the alley behind our Brooklyn townhomes. We hid behind drapes and peeked at her, giggling and mocking her disheveled gray hair and dirty clothes. As my stepfather threatened to leave me behind while the rest of the family moved to New Jersey, I wondered if the Crazy Old Baby Carriage Lady had been told to "shape up or ship out." I wondered if she had been left behind to a life of pushing a baby carriage and sifting through garbage. I couldn't get it out of my mind.

While my parents packed up the house, a distant aunt and uncle showed up to take me and my younger sister to stay with them. I was sure we were being shipped out, and they were only keeping my baby sister. My parents assured us that it was only temporary, and we would soon be in a nice big house in New Jersey – a house with a yard. I asked if we could get a horse. Everyone laughed.

The time with our aunt and uncle was pleasant, yet a bit odd. They had no children, and I don't think they knew what to do with us. My sister and I remained quiet and well-behaved; fearing that this would become our new permanent residence, I didn't want to do anything to get shipped out again.

It was a big relief when our parents came to fetch us, and we headed to New Jersey. But instead of a big house with a yard (for the horse), our car stopped in front of an odd-looking vehicle parked in an area that looked more like a junkyard than a new neighborhood. It wasn't a car or a truck, but it had wheels. It had windows. It had steps to get inside.

The trailer park was in Moonachie, New Jersey, squeezed onto a plot of land near the New Jersey Turnpike and huge belching oil refineries. The air was pungent. The trailers were lined up close to each other, and through a window, I could see the multiple cats prowling on the neighbor's window ledges. Occasionally, I would wander over to visit. The smell of cat pee was a change compared to the oil refinery smoke. It wasn't home, but I was at least with my family. It was summer, so enrolling in a new school wasn't worrisome. I didn't understand why we were there – the adult issues would only become clear years later when history repeated itself.

We moved into a house just in time to begin 5th grade. Minus the horse, this new state of farmland was everything I expected. To the outside world, we had it all: a lovely house, a manicured neighborhood, and nearby schools. Yet, the home held many secrets.

My mother became a widow when I was three weeks old. I have snippets of memories in which my mother was crying at night. The music she listened to became the backdrop of my babyhood – even years later, I would hear those tunes and feel sad without knowing why. She remarried when I was three years old, and I shouted to a packed subway car, "I have a Daddy now!" He was a Marine, like my deceased father, doing his best for my mom, me, and eventually for my two half-sisters.

Years later, I would understand his difficult upbringing after his father abandoned his wife and six children. His mother became a strict disciplinarian, even barring a pregnant, unmarried daughter from coming home until she gave the baby up. He also lived with the uncertainty of never knowing when they would have to move to a different dwelling. On her rare visits, his mother was still a scary woman.

In the New Jersey house, I knew little of my parents' trauma, only that there were large quantities of it, and my mother lost her soul to it. My stepfather, who truly loved my mother, gave in to her addiction, joined in at times, and lived with the belief that she had never recovered from the loss of my father, the reminder that made her so sad. Any hint of criticism of her would warrant swift punishment, including being held up in the air by my neck, which caused me to pass out and pee myself.

I didn't know my mother's alcoholism was partially rooted in home insecurity. As a young girl, she spent three years in a hospital for spinal fusion, and when she came home, there was no longer a bed for her. She was forced, at 14 years of age, to sleep in bed with her parents, and the shame caused by a drunken father mistaking her for his wife.

All I knew was that home was uncomfortable and scary. In those days, no one at school was interested in what was happening to kids "at home." A friend of mine was beaten so severely by a parent that she missed three weeks of school. Who could guess how many of my classmates were just waiting to get out of the house? The house was not a home. At age 18, poised for college, I was unable to hang on for just four more years as a commuter student living at home, engulfed in rising trauma. Home was no haven; I had to escape.

I left with nothing but the clothes on my back and whatever was in my pocketbook.

For all I knew, it was the start of me becoming the Crazy Old Baby Carriage Lady. I was terrified and panicked, but I would not return. No one came to look for me either, which cemented the idea that I had no home and hadn't all along.

My boyfriend's parents found me a room to rent. Police escorted me back to the house to get my clothes and personal belongings. As the officer chatted with my parents about ungrateful children, I entered a room I didn't recognize. It was completely trashed. Drawers dumped on the floor. Clothes torn from hangers. Anything that my parents thought they paid for was either gone or smashed. I could hear my sisters crying in the other room, just like my mother crying in her room so many years before. They were terrified to talk to me.

Over the following years, I had shelter but no home. I changed apartments several times and worked two jobs to pay the rent. Peanut butter was my staple. Again, friends helped me. I got a job at a large pharmaceutical company and was employed there for 10 years. By then, I was married, and we would eventually have three children.

We moved from an apartment into a house we built – and I thought, finally, a real home – a real family. My children would never go through what I went through. They would always have the stability I lacked and never fear being "shipped out" or "left behind." "Home Sweet Home" was not only shelter but a loving, safe, and secure environment.

And it was wonderful until it wasn't. The divorce agreement specified that the house be sold, and my teenagers and I faced finding a new place to live. I purchased a small townhouse, put my girls in one bedroom and my son in the other. I slept on a day bed in the partially finished basement.

The townhouse never became "home" as bills mounted, utilities were turned off, and the HOA was pounding on my door for its fees. Even with child support, we were four people trying to live on 50% of what five people had previously lived on. We were living paycheck to paycheck and still carrying a negative account.

I needed something more affordable, and the house hunt was agonizing. I found one a place with two small bedrooms, a much less appealing sort-of finished basement, and a lumpy, weedy yard unsuitable for a horse but great for the dog.

We packed up the townhouse, and the night before closing, I slept on the floor in a sleeping bag, snuggling with the dog. The kids were with their father for his weekend. Everything was in storage for two weeks so we could clean and paint. The budget was going to be more affordable. Things would calm down.

The next morning, my realtor called me. The closing was canceled. The person we were purchasing the house from had not disclosed that she was in bankruptcy and was trying to keep the court from knowing she had just inherited the house. The title company tracked it down. The sale was stopped. But the sale of the townhouse proceeded. Suddenly, we were homeless. Houseless. There was nowhere for me and the dog to go. I sat in my car – now my only shelter, hugged the dog and cried.

The second bit of bad news was that the seller had 30 days to rectify the bankruptcy, and during that time, I could not get back my deposit or purchase another house. The money from the townhouse sale was supposed to be used to fix up the next house. Finish the basement properly and add a bathroom. Instead, that money began slipping away for furniture storage fees, paying for an extended stay hotel room, and kenneling the dog. Thirty days passed, the bankruptcy was not rectified, and I was on the hunt again for a place to live.

Meanwhile, I was separated from my kids, lying awake at night in a strange place full of strange noises, shady people, and the sound of fire alarms blaring in the middle of the night. Even so, it didn't escape me that I was luckier than many others, especially after the local destruction of homes by Hurricane Floyd.

**I had a job, a car, and some money to keep me afloat.
For a while.**

In a familiar replay, summer ended, and there was no nice house or new school on the horizon. The kids were still staying with their father in another town. We decided that my oldest daughter would drive the three of them to the high school they had previously been attending and keep secret that we no longer lived in town. It was just a taste of what many homeless families go through to keep their kids in school – false addresses.

Non-custodial family members or friends often keep kids at their house for school days. I felt tremendous guilt asking my children to endure the anxiety this produced for them. I later realized that my actions could have gotten me arrested.

The only money I had left could pay for a HUD loan if I could find an affordable place in the same town. I gave up the extended stay hotel and camped at my sister's with her three teenagers. The entire time, I remained employed and paid taxes, yet my family was "homeless."

Finally, finally, I found something affordable. We all hated it – one bathroom, no air conditioning, and the heat was nearly nonexistent when needed, even in the tiny rooms. We had to go to the laundromat. Once more, I was sleeping on a day bed, but in the living room because there was only a crawl space, no basement. Only the dog seemed happy; after all, he was released from doggie jail and returned to a yard.

We managed – of course, there was constant bickering about bathroom time, especially in the morning. There was a continuous parade of repairs, including a scary burnout of wires under the house. Going to the laundromat was miserable. But little by little, the house began to resemble a home.

My son, perhaps because of his own experiences, had a group of friends we called "the lost boys," who, living in their own difficult situations, came over for dinner, stayed overnight, and one of them spent months with us to finish high school after his family moved away. I don't know if it was a shape-up or ship-out situation, but his parents moved, and he stayed.

In 2009, the recession hit. My entire award-winning department was eliminated in one fell swoop! I had never lost a job in my life. In fact, I always got any job I ever applied for, but the recession changed that. Unemployment did not cover the mortgage. Job applications went unanswered. The familiar feeling of bills piling up and collectors hounding me returned.

The small amount of money I had squirreled away in a retirement account disappeared, and I ended up owing taxes for the withdrawals. While I hadn't thought of her in years, the Crazy Old Baby Carriage Lady began to haunt me. I considered letting the bank take the house, and I'd just rent.

Then, I discovered that rental properties were not easy to come by. Landlords now ran credit checks and even required proof of income. With a foreclosure and a circling-the-drain credit score, I quickly realized there would be no rental. I finally found a new job, though for thousands less than I had been making. Foreclosure was still being threatened. I could hear the wheels of the baby carriage in my sleep.

At the last possible minute, banks relented, giving "underwater" homeowners like me a six-month reprieve to only pay interest. Of course, it lengthened the mortgage, but it provided a little bit of a lifeline. I am still in this house today, still making repairs when I can afford it. I found a loving partner I've been living with for 13 years and am grateful for the understanding and support he provides me when my childhood anxiety and sense of uncertainty raise their ugly heads.

I spent a good portion of my life afraid of being homeless. We are all one catastrophe, illness, job loss, or trauma away from becoming unsheltered. I'm grateful for the parts of my brain that continually remind me of how much worse things could be if I developed a substance-use disorder like my mother did.

I am also thankful to the Crazy Old Baby Carriage Lady – who was really just an unhoused person trying to survive – a person we mocked and laughed at because we didn't know better. In fact, this is the last time I will refer to the unhoused woman with that dreadful childish title. Going forward, she will remind me that everyone deserves a place to call home.

Feeling insecure about future living conditions is still a big issue for me. The statistics regarding unsheltered senior citizens are alarming. For those needing care, it is even more bleak. I am 68 years old, still have three jobs, and the anxiety is never far away.

Noreen Braman: *To Dale Ford, who helped me understand the real meaning of home.*

Can't We All Just Get Along

By Dr. Jo Anne White
My Conversation with Fred, Indianapolis,
Indiana, USA

Tap into the amazing riches within you.
They will see you through challenges and sorrows and pave
the way for a grateful today and new tomorrows.

Dr. Jo Anne White

*F*red Young was close to his mom. She was primarily responsible for her family of eleven children. Fred's father's life consisted of working long hours to support their large family, and he did so without complaints. Since his father always worked, Fred aimed to make his mother's life easier. With so many children to feed, teach, and help grow, he didn't want to be a burden to her.

This was one of the main reasons that Fred signed up for the military a few months before his eighteenth birthday. He was a Refueling Petroleum Supply Specialist and served three years active duty and another three years in the reserve. Alcohol and drug usage started at age thirteen. Fred drank because he was shy. Alcohol seemed to help his friends communicate easily, so he thought, why not me? He also started smoking marijuana around that time too.

In the military, Fred was introduced to hard drugs, and his reliance on them worsened. Alcohol and drugs were easy to acquire there, which intensified his addiction. It almost cost Fred his honorable discharge.

After the military, Fred worked at General Motors, a job he started in 1979. He was making good money. Yet the bills were piling up, and the money that was supposed to go to rent never made it. The money he earned went to drugs instead. His addictions got the better of him. That's when Fred lost housing, too.

No longer could he pay rent. Fred was losing control and felt that he had to quit or he would surely die. He reasoned that if he continued to work at General Motors, he wouldn't stop using drugs and would eventually OD. Additionally, he wanted to leave before he got fired due to missing too much work and failing numerous drug tests. So Fred walked away from the job.

With no apartment and no job, Fred was out on the street in Indianapolis for five long years and was homeless from 1995 until 2000. He had lost so much in the way of respect, family, friends, and even hope, but not his faith. Fred became part of a clique that bolstered him. Here, he felt he belonged and was connected to others, unsheltered like him, so the self-judgment wasn't so severe. For many people, that sense of comradery and of belonging can keep them unsheltered.

Not everyone is on the street due to drugs. Fred didn't realize until much later in his life, when he was in recovery, that he had mental health issues. He learned that he was deeply suffering from anxiety and depression.

Living under the bridge and sleeping in a refrigerator box became the norm. It was one way, maybe the only way at the time, not to be exposed to the elements. One evening, a truck entered the area. It was at that moment that the awareness set in. Fred realized that he could have been run over, dead in his sleep. This foreboding took hold, and he was shaken by the thought.

They often slept in vacant houses. One time, Fred left to go to church. When he returned, the house was ablaze. His two comrades were deeply agitated, thinking that Fred was in the house as the fire burned on incessantly.

Gangs began to jump on people living on the street, beating them up and setting them on fire. Often, they did it just for fun because the unsheltered were vulnerable and easy to attack. Sometimes, it was part of the initiation to become a standing gang member. It intensified over the years, which increased the fears of unsheltered individuals of being killed or physically harmed.

Being on the street was hard, especially when Fred had to beg for food or money. It often meant facing harsh judgment from others in their eyes, facial expressions, or words. What was worse was not even being seen. It was as if they didn't exist at all.

This made Fred look deeply at himself. He was later able to stay at the VA Harbor Light Mission Salvation Army. Beds were limited. Fred didn't know when he got there if all the beds would be occupied and he'd be left out again in the cold night. Someone asked him, "Did you pray on it?" He realized that he hadn't. He finally prayed, and thankfully, a bed was available when he arrived. Fred broke down in tears. Here was an opportunity to have a place to sleep, sheltered from the cold and from unwelcomed eyes or roaming predators.

At halfway houses, it was mandatory to take a breathalyzer test. You could be rejected due to drugs or alcohol. This made him take another hard look at himself. Fred realized that he couldn't go on this way forever. His so-called friends, street and drug buddies, didn't continue to hang around when his money was gone. He couldn't blame them. Isolated and feeling more alone, Fred thought it was up to him to somehow turn his life around. His determination to free himself from his addictions got even stronger.

Seeing so many more teens on the street was another shock and also an eye-opener for Fred. It gave him another reason to pull himself together, come off the street, and help others. "I have to work on myself every day. It's an ongoing process," says Fred. Even to this day, working on oneself is mandatory to stay ahead and be free of addiction.

You never know if being unsheltered can happen to you. It can happen in the blink of an eye. During the Covid shutdown, people came home and suddenly discovered they had lost their jobs. The glaring and unsettling truth set in when they realized they no longer had a way to support themselves. The large volume of evictions left many people experiencing homelessness. Many shelters were forced to reduce their capacity due to the coronavirus pandemic.

The stark reality is that people on the streets were and still are more likely to have health issues and be more susceptible to catching diseases. Unfortunately, since rent and mortgage rates are currently soaring and there has been a decline in coronavirus pandemic assistance, housing is out of reach for so many more Americans than previously.

"My journey back from a hopeless state of mind and body started at Pathway to Recovery," says Fred. Here was where he later sheltered and received support. At this time, working with people who were invested in his well-being and who taught him so much gave Fred the much-needed incentive, encouragement, and motivation to succeed.

More awareness set in. "I wanted to hold myself accountable while they held me accountable," Fred affirmed. For the people who worked there, it wasn't about the money. "You could feel the love; they truly cared. By the grace of God, this made a tremendous difference," Fred stated. When people's care and concern are genuine, you can feel it. It's uplifting and self-affirming.

Their caring and investment allowed Fred to be more self-invested and increased his desire to break the cycle of addictions. At Pathways, he chaired dual diagnosis meetings for a year, which bolstered his self-esteem.

Later, Fred moved into a house with three other people and worked at Sears. At that time, Sears received credit for hiring veterans. "Blessings again; they keep coming," he claimed. Despite pain, two hip replacements, and multiple surgeries that Fred has undergone, he sees his life now as a blessing.

Fred has been clean and sober for twenty-four years! Today, Fred works for HVAF: Helping Veterans and Families with "Hope,

Housing, and Self-Sufficiency For All Veterans And Their Families" to help them achieve the best possible quality of life. He's a peer mentor, *Community Health Worker (CHW), and Certified Recovery Specialist (CRS),* helping others who are or who have been unsheltered and/or suffering from addictions.

Fred has learned to listen and calls it "opening up doors." After they share, it leads him into more conversation, forming a true connection. Trust develops because they learn that he, too, was on the streets and was addicted to drugs and alcohol. Yet, with hard work on himself and seeking the necessary help, he overcame the addictions and chose to help others.

This turnaround can serve as a role model for others. "If Fred can do it, then maybe I have a chance, and I can do it too" can be a silent refrain and a strong motivator for others.

"When dealing with and supporting people with addictive and mental health issues, I can't just say all you have to do is try," declares Fred.

Mental health is much more complicated than that. There's a lot that's involved with mental health and even addiction that aren't visible. No one situation can be alike. The dialogue and understanding of mental health challenges are better than they were previously, but still not enough. There's stigma related to mental health as well as to being unsheltered.

Mental health and being unsheltered are often tied together. If the person experiencing both isn't aware, as in Fred's situation, it can still be challenging, especially without the right support and treatment. Fred chose to get the help and treatment that truly saved his life. His commitment to bettering himself is a lifelong one now. Fred's faith and commitment to God is strong. "I acknowledge God for his guidance and direction," Fred affirms.

We all need to have an ongoing commitment to ourselves, to our health, and our mental and emotional well-being. When we ignore our challenges and turn a blind eye to others with mental health issues or who've been unsheltered, we not only do them a disservice, we do ourselves a disservice as well.

When Fred was in grade school, a teacher asked him what he wished for. "I wish everybody could get along, smile, and be happy," answered Fred. We're not there yet, especially if we don't tackle the misunderstanding, stigma, and judgments surrounding being unsheltered and mental health. What's needed for people who are or have been unsheltered is first for others to truly listen and attempt to understand. They need to be given a chance, which can make all the difference. Today, more than ever, we have an opportunity to do that. Maybe when we do, we'll be more equipped and ready to smile, and all get along.

Dr. Jo Anne White ~ *My appreciation and gratitude go out to Fred Young for having the courage and authenticity to share his story of being unsheltered and for his continuous, unfailing support of others.*

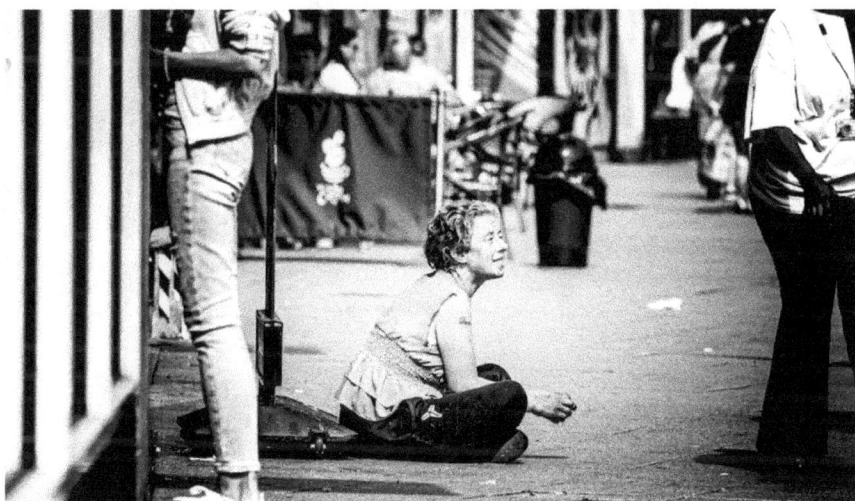

United Kingdom
Sarah Harvey, Photographer

Being Homeless – Homeless Being

By Patricia McNair
Atlantic, Canada

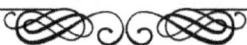

꧁꧂

*H*ow many times a day, week, or even a month does the average person even think of the fact that there are millions of homeless people all over the world? Does one think of it just out of the blue while baking cookies? Perhaps, but unlikely.

What does one think of while taking a warm crystal healing bath – maybe in the passing of a prayer or wish for All in need? What about seeing the homeless on a street while walking to the shops?

Let's take a walk and see how people react to the Homeless. Here we are, look. Do you see it? Yup, some are walking with their eyes closed until they can get by them ... just a few more steps and AHH, yes – invisible to the consciousness.

Look, some sneering and ignoring them as if they were nothing! I knew I would be able to show you those. "What can I get you? Here is $50.00. Can I video this – my social media followers will love that I am so kind – YES!"

Homeless. Close your eyes if you dare and say that word a few times. What tone, emotion, or thought comes up for you? Keep saying it. Could you say it more than five times? No? Are you brave enough to try it again in a week? Maybe getting past the "I don't want to think about it. It has nothing to do with me" or whatever you came up with to pass by the uneasiness of the word as quickly as possible.

If you felt defensive, were you able to move into a loving place?

What were you triggered to think or take action? Pray or maybe reach out with kind thoughts? Did you get to a place where you felt you could be of service in some small way? Awesome!

Even though that warm fuzzy emotional part may come through for someone reading this story, it is not remotely about that. I simply asked you to step into what the word homeless stirred up in you – well done. Either way, it transformed you. I am grateful that we could share that tiny experience together. Now, like I always say, "Let's go deeper."

There are many varieties of homelessness. I didn't say a variety of reasons for homelessness – of which there are. I said many varieties. Please let me explain it in my way as I have lived a few varieties of homelessness in my life.

Born and not Taken Home

As a baby, when I was not in the hospital for one reason or another, I was taken – not "home," but to any neighbor who would take me in. My mom would, ahem, visit once in a while, but she did not want to take me home. When I got healthier and became stronger, and there was no need for me to frequent the hospital, my so-called "visits" with different neighbors became longer and more strained.

As I grew and time quickly passed, those in my life became a bit blurry, and I still did not have a "home."

I remember when I was about 3.5 years old, my older brother and I had been staying with a really good friend of our mom's for a while. Mom came and spent the night! Yay! She tickled us, we laughed and even got a bath with some nice smelly soap. She tucked us in. WOW! I remember falling asleep and feeling loved by my mom. I thought, "I bet she is going to take us home tomorrow, and I will know where I belong and not be a lil' girl without a Home any longer."

The next day, I was so excited to wake up. I sang and danced in the living room. Mom dressed me and my brother in new, really pretty clothes. I heard a car pull up and ran to the window – only to see my mom talking to a tall man – and putting what looked like two big paper bags of mine and my brother's clothes in the trunk. I wanted to stay excited. Really, I did.

But something didn't feel right. The tall man and my mom came into the house, and she told us he would take my brother and me out for ice cream. What? Everything inside of me exploded. I started yelling, "No, he is not – you put our clothes in the trunk – we are not coming back. We are going to be homeless all our lives!"

Moved Around a lot of Homes – Not Home

Sure enough, we were being taken to a foster home. This was the first foster home of many. After a while, my brother went to live with an aunt, and I was placed into home after home. Foster homes were never real homes. Not my HOME. And most of them let you know the difference.

Finally Home – Homeless at Home.

At the ripe age of twelve, a judge forced me into the care of my mom. Not in any way what I wanted. The few visits I had with her over the years had always consisted of alcoholic boyfriends abusing her and her screaming about how much she hated me. Though the judge knew better, I had no say.

When she picked me up, she clarified that she did not want to have me back and that the situation was probation, only temporary, and if I didn't toe the line, she would see that I got placed in a home for girls. So, I did get to "go home" with my mom, but it made no difference. I was homeless there, too.

After a lot of abuse in unimaginable ways and things that happened that do not fit in this story, I ran away to the streets.

Homeless by My Choice and Scared out of My Wits!

At first, I hid so she couldn't find me. What was I thinking? After a short while, I knew she would not even bother.

During that time of my life, I would stay with different friends at their places off and on but would usually retreat to my old, abandoned car behind a garage that had gone out of business. I worked and could barely live off of my earnings. I liked knowing I had that car to go to when people would start catching on and asking too many questions about my family or where I lived.

Some horrific things happened, so I moved to the big city – it was definitely solace from where I came from. There were many homeless people there, and they all had their clicks and ways. I was terrified, to say the least.

Homeless with Help!

A few weeks later, I was approached and offered a spot to stay at a homeless shelter. Once again – now even the title said it all.

I got a job as a caregiver for a company in the city, and the homeless shelter gave me bus tickets to get to work. I met a friend at work, and she seemed so nice and caring. She thought I had beauty. She was caring, alright. She invited me to a celebration dinner. We went and got new dresses and got our hair done – the whole shebang.

I remember drinking a glass of what they all said was expensive wine and then waking up in the back seat of a car where two very large men were doing white powders. They were taking me to a bigger city to sell me. I was given the choice to smoke or snort this powder, or they would put it in a needle. Something told me I would NOT survive if it were a needle.

Homeless and Desperate to Survive

For over a year and a half, I ran for my life, living on the streets from big city to big city until I broke away and returned to my little town. I tried to share what had happened to me, but no one believed me. So, I stopped sharing and tried my best to blend in to try to have friends. I even got married. I was extremely self-aware, yet nothing felt real; I did not fit in. Life continued, and so many things happened: divorce, terminal illness, and heartbreak on so many levels.

I was Homeless by choice, and it felt like FREEDOM.

I wanted to be alone now! I needed to heal. I wanted to BE ME. I packed some sacred things in my little car, and I drove and drove and drove. I drove right out of Canada. I asked my friends to sell my belongings a piece at a time to buy gas and basic foods. I cried. I starved. I ate. I laughed and was happy yet so freaking unhappy all at once. I cried out to the Creator, and I yelled at myself for things that were not even my fault.

I did some massive healing and self-truth, recognizing and gaining my self-worth – releasing untruths, shame, blame, and guilt. Up to that point, it was the most empowering time of my life.

HOME at Last!

I found myself, stood in my holy light, and my heart flowed open to All that I am Universally. The Creator guided me to my true soul mate, to whom I have been happily married for over 22 years. We purchased our home, and we live happily in it today.

I am so happy that I was brave enough to Be Homeless by choice and allow myself the Freedom to BE. As I shared in my story, I have experienced many varieties of homelessness.

For centuries, many cultures did not have homes. Many were nomads traveling the land and setting up camps. The big difference then, perhaps in the Community, was the Home. The family. The glue. I have thought about this so many times. While I have experienced traumatic varieties of homelessness, I have also had beautiful achievements and solace while being homeless.

I tip my hat to any homeless person. The reason or circumstances in which they are homeless is between them and the Creator.

When thinking of fellow homeless brothers and sisters, two common sayings always come to mind. Even thirty years ago, it was a saying, "Most people are only one paycheck away from being homeless." Have you seen major improvements over the last thirty years? Hasn't it been the rich getting richer and the poor getting poorer? Seriously, how could that mantra remotely touch the issue of people being homeless?

Also, the common saying of "Home Is Where Your Heart Is."

So, the next time you look at a homeless brother or sister, try to look past the tattered clothes, dirty face, or the position in which they are sitting, standing, or walking. Look past what society proclaims as success and yet does everything to take away one's value, dignity, and wellbeing. With your heart, look at this child of the Creator, and look into their heart.

WHERE IS THEIR HEART LIVING? Despair, conquered, alone, confused, low self-worth, or lost? Why might their heart be living there? Being respectful, ask questions, and get to know them. What's their story? Ask how you could assist them. For only a few minutes of your day, show them human connection and kindness. You can do volumes more with this approach rather than trying to fix them or their situation. Are you truly more successful and better than them – because you have…?

Connecting with homeless people will be a gift, opportunity, and choice to be human. Try not to judge or shun them; come full circle by becoming more open and aware of how a brother or sister has found themselves in that space. Welcome to your homelessness experience!

Patricia McNair ~ *I thank the Loving Creator, Spirit, My Divine Being, as well as my wonderful partner, Patrick, and our lil man, Q. Many thanks go out to All in Oneness in my life so far—the positive and not-so-positive. All matters in who and what I stand in as I reach out for every step to do my part in the Divine Plan. Thank You.*

Interview with Mark Harpur

Southampton, England

By Dennis Pitocco

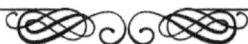

‿‿‿

*T*ell me about your homeless experience, Mark.
It all began when I left home at 17, and it was because of a mixture of things. I don't really want to go into the reasons too much, but...

Where was home?
My home was Belfast. Basically, what happened was that home life wasn't great. I had three sisters, two of whom … I don't know if this is for the book, so I won't name names, but two of whom had been taken into care.

It was difficult because my dad was bringing up four kids on his own in a very – I don't know whether I would say a religious society – but I would say a very conservative society. One of the first families that I knew of that had got divorced.

My mother wanted to take two of us to Australia, of which one wasn't me. I never knew my mom, and I met her for the first time at my youngest sister's funeral. So, that's sort of where all of that kind of ties in. But I'm happy to talk about it.

I have some questions for you that might make it a little clearer. You said you were 17, and you were on the streets of Belfast?
Um, no. I moved out of the family home and got on a boat to Scotland only because that was all I could afford.

Why did you move out of the family home?
I would say it was a combination of things. It was a breakdown in communication.

So you felt it was best for you. Was it your choice to move out because of your own wellbeing?
Yeah, it was. It was bad. You could put it like that. I mean, I could go deeper than that.

And you said you moved onto the streets of Belfast, but you went to Scotland. So, were you on the streets of Belfast?
I wasn't on the streets of Belfast at all. I got a ferry on a Friday evening to Scotland and hitched from Stranraer, a ferry port in Scotland.

So, the ferry went from a place called Lorne, and that's about 18 miles outside Belfast. And I got the train down to Lorne. Got the ferry across to Stranraer in Scotland, and I hitchhiked all the way to a district in Glasgow called White Craig's. From there, I walked into roughly what was the city center.

It was about a seven-mile walk. At one stage, I was fairly good on my legs, but obviously, the impact of the disability, getting older, and putting on a few pounds probably contributed to where I am now. But just to say, I walked into the city center, where a train station was on Hope Street.

I went there initially, and then I met a fella who'd just recently moved to his own flat, but he'd been homeless about two or three months previous. And he showed me a bench in a park in central Glasgow surrounded by foliage.

So I slept there for a night, and then because I didn't know how to make connections with things – you know, I was pretty green behind the ears – the next day, I went to a soup kitchen run by the Salian, which is the Salvation Army in a district in Glasgow called Denison. They kind of fed and watered me for a while.

Was that housing of some kind?
No, it wasn't. No, at this stage, it wasn't any kind of housing.

So it was just food?
Yeah, just basically food.

So, you would spend every day walking the streets of Glasgow, and then you would go there for food?
Yeah.

How long were you on the streets in Glasgow?
I had two periods where I was homeless. And they were actually in quick succession. I was on the street for probably three or four weeks.

And then I got into the system, so to speak because I had spoken to somebody from the Salvation Army, and they told me, "Well, you could go down to a hotel on Duke Street."' It was called the Great Eastern or the Great Western. I have a funny feeling it was the Great Eastern.

It's been pulled down now, but it used to have rooms that were very, very little and... I don't know how you would describe them, but basically, you had people there. It was a controlled environment in that you had a reception and people on the door.

And a place to sleep?
And a place to sleep, yeah.

So, when you were staying at the hostel and had to be out from 10 o'clock until about three or four in the afternoon, how did you then spend your day?
So, a lot of the time, I used to go to the Salvation Army and help them set up. I thought to myself, "Well, I found myself in this predicament, the least I can do is help out." So I did that. They used to get a lot of clothes, so I used to go up there, you know, probably from the time that we were meant to leave at 10 o'clock.

Did you have any source of income at all/any kind of government assistance?
No, not at that point. I did, obviously, later on. Basically, the problem that you have is that initially, you would have to have a permanent address.

And while the state would pay for your bed and breakfast at the hostel because they knew you're staying there, they also knew that that's not really a permanent address, if you understand what I mean.

So, they would pay for that sort of thing, but in terms of money, not really. I think the system's changed a bit now, but at the time, that wasn't the case. So that's one of the reasons why I used to go and help set up with the Sally Army.

And rather than doing the food, I would sort through the clothes that they would get. And obviously, that'd make them available for me.

When you were actually on the street, Mark, did you feel safe?
I did, but as I said, the first period in Glasgow, not so much. Funnily enough, not so much. But I was homeless for the second time in London, and that felt much more so.

What was your biggest fear on the streets?
Being attacked by other homeless people or the public if, on an odd occasion, I had decided to sleep in a doorway.

So your first time homeless, you were staying in a hostel for a while and getting some help, and then you got off the street briefly before returning?
Yeah, so what happened was Glasgow City Council, through their housing stocks, offered me a flat. And I thought it would be a good opportunity.

It just, from the get-go, descended into something bad, you know. I thought I was going to be able to make something of it, but what happened was it was all a housing scheme called Drumchapel in Glasgow. Slightly naive, I went to view the place. They had mesh wiring up rather than windows. They told me I could have it, and I was grateful.

And I suppose I didn't really know what I was getting myself into. So I said, right, I'll take it. But what happened was I had a friend come and visit me over Christmas and New Year's. On New Year's, we decided to go and have a drink to celebrate, you know, Hog, the Scots call it Hogmanay. We went out, and when we were out, we met this lad called Danny. Basically, I would say we befriended him.

This guy, Eddie, turned up at my front door, and I didn't know how he found out where I was living; well, I found out later that he didn't live that far away, but somehow, he found out where I was living. Basically, he knocked on my door one day and told me that my older sister, Edith, was being kicked out of the house by our parents.

At the time, it was a two-bed place, right?
Yes, and he asked me, would you be prepared to let her stay with you for a while until she gets sorted out? And, of course, having just been through what I went through, I thought it would be ungracious of me not to try and help her.

And, so I said, fair enough, and basically that night, I got a knock on the door. There were about 20 people at the door. I didn't know at the time that there were 20 people. I opened the door, and these people just came rushing into the front. It was a complete age range. In fact, I found out that one of the fellas in the group actually lived above me with his father. That was upsetting because, out of the group of people that came in, Chris, his name was, probably had a little bit of fun with me because he knew what was happening, but obviously, I didn't know what was happening.

But by this stage, I was working as a jeweler in Enoch Square in Glasgow. And as I say, when they come in, they follow the leader. I would describe him as Fagin from the *Oliver Twist* story because obviously, he was the leader. He used to get the people that were there. They didn't all stay there, by the way, because they had homes to go to, but of a normal night, you would have about 10 of them staying.

So, we came to a mutual understanding that my bedroom, to anybody, was off-limits. Well, you'd be just kidding. Because I thought to myself, what did I do? I didn't feel like I could go to the police because I thought I'd get beat up if I did that. You know, this was the thing, and when I used to go to work, two of them used to come and sort of keep an eye out to make sure I wasn't saying anything. I know it sounds absolutely nuts, but basically, this guy Andrew used to send them out to rob people or steal stuff from the department stores, all that kind of thing.

They were using the homeless people to become their network of thieves.

Yeah. They were all from the local Drum Chapel area. The Chapel was probably about six miles outside Glasgow. But, of a morning, he'd send them out, and some of them might go to Annie's Land, but the bulk of them would go into Glasgow Centre, so the likes of Suckery, Old Street, and places like that. And they would come back with their ill-gotten gains from the day, so basically the shoplift, and go back to him. I suppose I'd describe him as a fence because he'd be able to sell it on to somebody.

Just to confirm, was it the second time you were homeless?
Yeah.

And that was about three weeks, and then you moved into the property?
Yeah, moved in.

How long did you stay there?
I was there until the second week of January. I moved in early, probably back at the end of October or early November. I wasn't there that long.

And then at that point, you went back onto the street?
My big idea was that I needed to get out of this situation.

As I said to you previously, we had an understanding that coming into my bedroom was off-limits. On the weekends, right? I mean, this was what they were up to. I tended to keep to myself, but they used to get high on the weekends.

I would say that there were probably taking Es [Ecstasy], which was pretty popular at the time, and stuff like that. Anyway, what happened was, one of them came into my bedroom, and I thought he was coming in to attack me, so I picked something up, hit him over the head with it – well, it was a plate – but he was basically coming to get a bit of weed that I had behind the bed.

Obviously, we fought, but the next thing I remember was waking up in Glasgow infirmary. As soon as they discharged me from there, I just had it in my head that I had to get away.

You were in the hospital/infirmary. They were taking care of you, and they were going to discharge you, and you really don't have a home. Did they just discharge you onto the street?
No, I still had the key for the flat, but by this stage, they had obviously got keys for the flat, so there was always a risk involved in going back. So I went back on the Thursday. And on the Saturday, I woke up at about half seven. They were doing drugs the night before, so they were basically everywhere in my place.

You made the decision it was time to leave?
Yeah, and I got on the bus back into Glasgow. Do you remember at the time they used to have the advertising on the bus saying ""Glasgow Smiles Better?"" And I used to think to myself, "'Does it?" Hell, it's just as bad as living in Belfast!

And anyway, because part of me thought to myself when I moved there, I thought, "I've jumped from the frying pan into the fire here."

When you got on the bus – at that point, you were homeless again?
Yeah, effectively. I got on the bus, and I got down to Buchanan Street, which was where the bus station was.

Oh, by the way, the address I lived at was Inchford Drive, in Drumchapel. So when the boss gets into the coach and then gets off, the boss walks to the coach station in Buchanan Street and buys a one-way ticket to London.

That's how you ended up in London?
I always remember the woman clerk said to me, and obviously she didn't know a lot of people through it, and she said to me, "'It's not a return," and I said, "No, no chance."

"Ah, good for you."

This sounds really stupid, but I thought I would go to London because I knew that my sister worked at Terminal 4 in Heathrow. She used to take care of a lot of the sort of Arab businessmen that were flying. They'd come to the kind of desk that she worked at, and she would set them up with taxis or cars or VIP cars or whatever it would be and set up accommodation for them if that was needed.

What eventually ended up happening was I got down there, to Heathrow, to try and find her, and this was on Saturday, but I couldn't find her. I thought to myself, "It's the weekend." I was sort of thinking it might be a nine-to-five job Monday to Friday with the weekends off, so, with that, I thought I might as well sleep in the terminal. So, I went to gate 48 to 50, Terminal 1.

On the tube, you can go from Terminal 4 and then back to Terminals 1, 2, and 3, right? And so I went back to Terminal 1. If anybody asked me, I'd say I missed the last flight back to Belfast. But, the next morning, a policeman saw me, and he was watching me. Obviously, I wasn't moving anywhere because this was on a Sunday, right? And I've obviously, at that stage, come to the conclusion that my sister probably wasn't working on a Sunday. I thought, "Should I move or should I not?" Anyway, with that, he came over and told me that if I didn't move on, he was going to arrest me for vagrancy.

So, that forced my hand. I had heard of Cardboard City, a kind of area between the Waterloo train station and the embankment. It was like an underpass.

Effectively, at its height, it had around 250-300 homeless people. And the reason why they called it Cardboard City was because of the amount of people creating their own personal space, but obviously, it's cardboard and sort of sleeping and stuff like that there.

So I went there and, like you asked me about Glasgow, did it feel safe doing that? I felt safer in Glasgow than I did when I was in Cardboard City. I was lucky enough to befriend two people, both of whom had alcohol problems, but they only really had alcohol problems for about 48 hours because they would spend what money they would get on alcohol, then when the money ran out, obviously, they're sober.

When you were living in Cardboard City, did the homeless people look after each other?
To an extent. You've got to remember that you're talking 1986, '87, right? So, by that stage, they were closing down the hospitals, or the asylums, if

you want to call it that. Some of those people were being catered for, for them to go out into the community.

But then there were some of that kind of people that got left behind. And, of course, those that got left behind ended up on the street. So you had people who had alcohol problems, drug addiction, marriage breakdown, runaways, a bit like me. You know, home life wasn't great.

The other thing I've got to say as well, Dennis [interviewer], is it wasn't just home life. I didn't enjoy growing up during the Troubles. Of course, I didn't understand people's thinking. It's like the beauty about being disabled because I went to a disabled school. The beauty of being disabled is it doesn't discriminate.

What is your disability?
I've got cerebral palsy.

And back when you talked about being homeless in 1986 in that area when you were in your teens, you weren't in a wheelchair yet?
No.

During this entire period of time, we're talking about back then when you were in Cardboard City, you were still in your teens, right?
Yeah.

How did the public treat you? Did you encounter the public much?
Like I was invisible.

It's more about human interaction and being recognized as a person. I mean, I think the thing is people realized that there was a problem, especially in and around that district where Cardboard City was. I think the people tolerated it.

I think one of the things that's important to say is this was kind of at the same time as *The Big Issue*. You've heard of the homeless magazine,

The Big Issue, right? So this would have been at the time when all this was kind of launching.

And obviously, the idea of *The Big Issue* is to give you the wherewithal to be able to push yourself forward kind of thing, and, obviously, then it helps people get housing and get settled in the settled routine if that's what they want. But I found that people struggle with the idea of having a home after they've spent a while on the street. I think there is this thing where if you end up on the street for too long, and I realized this fairly early, it can have a real kind of psychological effect on people.

And during that time period, when you were on the street and involved in Cardboard City, how long was it before you finally moved off the street again?

That would have been maybe January. There was a soup kitchen that was done by a group called Helping Hands, who, ironically, were a bunch of Franciscan monks based in East London. They eventually ended up taking me in, and they lived at 42 Ballam Street. The place is still there, and the head Franciscan monk is still there. Julian. It's amazing. Julian and they were really, really good people to me. I can't speak highly enough about my friends.

So they were responsible for you finally coming off the street and transitioning back into the mainstream, for lack of a better term?

Yeah. There was a brother called Brother Silas. And effectively, he used to come, basically, to do the soup kitchen with one or two others. After getting to know me a little, he said, "Why don't you come and stay in the house with us for a bit?" And obviously, I'm a little bit doubtful because I'm sort of sitting there thinking, "Yeah, but you're kind of like an enclosed community because you're talking about people that walk around with the food and monkey around."

It works, you know. And they're out in the community. I used to find it really strange because there was a guy that was from Kent, and he loved Israel. And you know, we would always go out and have two pints together every week. He'd buy a pint, and I'd buy a pint.

He loved Kentish beer and Shepherd Mead, and I used to get some strange looks when I was out in the pub with about three or four of the monks, all in their habits. But yeah, it was good times, and that did help me because I ended up doing a bit of volunteering for them.

This sounds ironic, but what I did was fill out supplementary benefit forms. This was in the East End of London in the Bangladeshi community that had come over to settle in London. And I was filling them out for the older members of the family – dare I say the parents or the grandparents – whose first language was not in English. So we'd go to the home, and I'd fill the form out. And then we'd go back to the Helping Hands office that had the Franciscan Brothers, and obviously, they would send it off.

So I did quite a bit of that, and then I went to work for the Home Office at St. Ann's Gate, and I got into the Civil Service.

How many years have you been off the street now?
I was 55 last week, so I've been off the streets for around 38 years now.

If you can look back at your time on the streets, what was the worst part?
The worst part was being frightened by the unknown, and a lot of the unknown was, dare I say, other homeless people because you couldn't predict them. Because of the different problems people had, you know, you had drug addictions, you had alcoholism, you had people whose marriages had broken down, you had runaway kids, and sometimes things would, especially in Cardboard City where there were so many people, things would tend to kick off, and I would feel vulnerable then.

I'd be sort of sitting there thinking that I didn't feel particularly safe, but eventually, it would all kind of die down, but it did happen quite regularly, like at least twice a week.

And it usually happened when people had money. When they didn't have money, it was more sort of harmonious because people weren't necessarily feeding. You know, I'm just talking from an addiction point of view, but people didn't necessarily have the money to feed the addiction. So they were having the return to normality.

A few days before, they would get their money again to do whatever it was that they were doing, and I used to find that sort of frightening within the homeless community. But I look back at it as something that I've experienced. I didn't particularly want to experience it, but I'm glad that I did.

Because it just made me realize that everybody's got a stake in society. And it doesn't matter where you're coming from or where you're necessarily going. And when you're on the street, you aren't really visible to people.

But I do think that's kind of changed over the years as well. I do think people, by and large, tend to engage, but then you can get the other side of the spectrum where people want to beat you up or whatever, just for being homeless. So it's a difficult one, but the realization for me was that I just, on both occasions, needed to get myself off the street here as quickly as possible.

You ultimately did that and should be pretty proud of yourself for how far you've come.
Yeah, it helps that I ended up in the South. I used to come over here on summer holidays. We had 10 weeks during the summer because my dad obviously remarried, and I look at her as being my mum; that's as simple as that.

So my grandmother and grandfather lived in Winchester, Oxford Road, and I would stay with them for a couple of weeks. But when my uncle used to phone, this is my uncle Tony, he'd say, "Mark, do you want to come down to Southampton for seven or eight weeks of the holiday?" I used to jump at the chance because he worked for the *Daily Echo* local paper.

He was a compositor for the *Daily Echo*, and I used to spend the summers basically helping him. And I loved going up to the news and sports desks, but that's a completely different thing. So, it sort of came full circle by my uncle Han.

You know, he has four children. One of them, David, committed suicide. I got back in touch with Han, and he suggested, "Why don't you move down to Southampton. I just like the idea of you being nearby."

And the thing is, when we'd come to Southampton or Winchester, I always felt loved and part of the family. So, since he basically asked me to consider moving down to Southampton, that's what I did.

You said you didn't have much of a relationship with your parents. Are either one of them still alive?
My dad died during the first lockdown.

Was that COVID-related or not?
No, no, stroke.

Did you have a chance to see him since your days on the street?
Yeah, I used to go back. It's not like I cut all ties. I didn't feel like I could do that. It was a really difficult relationship, but I always looked at it as, with my mom being the way she was, and she didn't really want anything to do with me, and my dad was bringing us up on his own, so I recognize that had its own pressures.

I used to go because Dad used to live in the family home still in Whitehead because Christine, she's still alive. Yeah, he died during COVID. My natural mother, I think she's still alive. She lives in a place called Ballyclare.

Have you stayed in touch with your sister, who used to work at Heathrow?
Yeah, when the lockdown was on, we did sort of speak. I've got to be honest, Dennis, because the girls were all older than me and were all very close, I always felt outside of that, so it's difficult. I still think I'm scarred by my childhood. And they don't want to talk about it. You know, that's basically their rule of thumb. You keep it in-house; you don't talk about it. I find benefit from talking about it. And I made the mistake of speaking to one of my eldest sister's daughter about it during lockdown. She just closed down again. Basically, she told me she didn't want anything to do with me.

Where do you live today?
I live in a district called Thornhill. It's on the east side of Southampton.

And you're settled there a while?

Yeah, but I've lived here in Southampton since 1995 or '96. Originally, it was in private accommodation, and I had a rent agreement, so it was a 10-year lease. But after the fifth year, they doubled the rent, and I thought, "Well, I'm not going to be able to pay for that." So, I went down to Southampton City Council, and thankfully, I still had the agreement and the rent schedule on the back. They recognized what the problem was because they said, "Well, you're not earning enough, and you're not getting enough from us to be able to cover it." So they offered me this place, and I've been here ever since. I moved here in 2002.

If you bumped into somebody today and you were out and about, Mark, and encountered a homeless person, would you offer them any wisdom, advice, guidance, or anything they should be doing if they're living on the street and feel helpless? You obviously figured out how to get off the street.

Yeah, and it took a while for the penny to drop in the sense that I was fortunate that there were one or two homeless people that I came into contact with in both cities that were able to give me advice about go to this soup kitchen or go here.

You know, I'll give you some sort of accommodation or roof over your head to start off with, and then you need to sort of build up from there. From there you can probably meet people and maybe make the kind of contacts you made.

Yeah, exactly. There are people that will help.

What was the hardest thing about being homeless?

The feeling of having no short-term security during my homeless period on the streets.

What did you learn from your time on the streets?

I will always try to help others when I can, especially in the disabled community, and not judge people.

What three words would you use to describe being homeless?

Invisible. Disconnected. Vulnerable.

Breaking the Chain:

A Glimpse into the Heart of Addiction and the Power of Hope

By Thea Nelson
USA

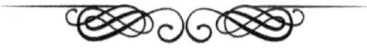

*For I know the plans I have for you, declares
the LORD, plans to prosper you and not to harm you,
plans to give you hope and a future.*

Jeremiah 29:11 NIV

*E*very city tells a story – tales of joy, love, and the darker side where addiction casts a long shadow. Read one family's encounter with the ruthless cycle of substance abuse, as witnessed through the harrowing experiences of a beloved niece. Journey from the suffocating depths of addiction, shaped by societal pressures and personal trauma, to the illuminating power of community and hope. Discover the devastating ripples of addiction, from shattered relationships to the profound loss of her firstborn. Yet, amidst the despair, stories of resilience, redemption, and humans' indomitable spirit emerge.

Recognizing addiction as more than a mere choice but as a complex interplay of emotions and circumstances, this story underlines the urgent need for compassion, understanding, and collective action. From personal tribulations to societal initiatives, we can break the chains of addiction and usher in a brighter, hopeful tomorrow. Join the movement, be the change, and together, we can rewrite the narrative for countless souls trapped in the vicious cycle.

Every city, whether small or large, has its stories. They paint pictures of joy, love, challenges, and, sometimes, the crippling grip of addiction. It's a topic intertwined in countless tales of those without a roof over their heads. Substance abuse, often seen as a shadowy figure lurking behind many homeless narratives, presents a challenge that's both heart-wrenching and eye-opening. Through a deeply personal lens, having witnessed one of my nieces grapple with addiction, I've come to see just how profound and heart-wrenching these stories can be.

A Descent into Darkness: The Why Behind the Slide

Imagine, for a moment, the weight of life pressing down on you. Financial hardships, loss, trauma, or societal pressures can create an overwhelming urge to escape. For some, that escape is found in substance abuse.

Life, with its unpredictable twists and turns, sometimes lands crushing blows. These challenges often drive individuals to seek refuge in drugs or alcohol. It began like that for my niece – a temporary escape from life's trials. A desire to fit in, the fever pitch of her anxiety, and the loss of her grandfather – the only father figure in her life. The alarming reality hit when this escape turned into multiple DUIs, a testament to addiction's worsening grip on her.

The darkest moment? She vanished for three days after an arrest in a different county. She didn't call for help due to embarrassment and fear, choosing to endure the isolation instead.

A Heartrending Search

When my niece went missing, it sent shockwaves through our family. We were frantic, looking everywhere for her. It felt like we were just a step away from calling everyone we knew to form a search party. And then, after three seemingly endless days, she turned up. The hardest part to digest? She had been locked up not far from us. It wasn't just a matter of her being gone; it was the unbearable thought that she was so close, yet we felt powerless.

Now, here's where the story takes a twist. The things people turn to for relief – drugs and alcohol – end up chaining them down. It's a cruel irony. It's not simply making a choice; it's a maze of feelings, body responses, and societal pressures.

Returning and reflecting on that time, the emotions come flooding back. Those three days were filled with panic, anxiety, and an overwhelming sense of hopelessness. But amidst all that, there was a silver lining. I discovered a strength I never knew existed within myself and our family. We realized the importance of leaning on one another, the incredible power of community, and the often-overlooked value of keeping faith and hope alive.

You might wonder if it's because I've watched one too many episodes of *Dateline* or *Unsolved Mysteries*, but when I learned she had been missing for a full day before we even knew? Well, it set off alarm bells. Suddenly, our 72-hour critical period shrank to just 48 hours. And honestly? My eyes were on her boyfriend.

You might be thinking, "Did you call the police?" We did. But they told us to hold tight, considering her age and some of her past behaviors.

The police may have wanted us to hold tight, but our family went into full action mode. People paired up, calling hospitals, county jails – even the coroner's office. And trust me: There's nothing more gut-wrenching than asking a coroner if they have an unidentified female. Every fiber of your being hopes for a "No." The last thing anyone wants to hear is "Yes" and have to describe the person they are looking for. They don't want to hear about the positive qualities of their loved one; they want factual details like height, weight, age, eye and hair color, build, scars, tattoos, etc. That's a hard call to make and a hard call to remember!

We did everything. We checked impound lots for her car and contacted her old and new friends. We called friends she hadn't been in contact with for years, in and out of state. I even visited places she frequented, showing her pictures, and asking if anyone had seen her.

We looked into nearby homeless shelters and kept an eye on her Facebook account, praying for any new activity. Thanks to a journalist friend, we even thought of getting the media involved at one point.

But then, just when things seemed bleakest, we found her. Or rather, she found her way home.

As much as I'd like to tell you this was some heartwarming movie reunion – it wasn't. It was emotionally charged, with everyone's anxiety levels cranked up. The joy of her return quickly shifted from a lost sheep returning to the herd to pressing questions about her whereabouts and actions.

I often wonder what was tougher for her: those three days she was away or facing the family's interrogation once she was back.

From all this, I've learned to live in the present, cherish moments more, empathize deeply, and be there for my family and friends quickly. I've also seen how vital it is to lend a hand to others, no matter how small the gesture. Because while the gesture seems small to me, it could be life-saving to the one receiving it.

Those three days felt like an eternity, and the realization that she had been locked up, so close yet so distant, was a wake-up call for all of us.

The cruel irony of this story? The mechanism sought for relief, the addiction, becomes the chain, anchoring so many to the streets, making the burden heavy on family and friends. And the addict is unaware of this weight.

Each addict is like a stone dropped in a pond, creating ripples. Their family and friends are those ripples, deeply affected and intertwined with the addiction. They often feel as powerless to aid the addict as the addict feels trapped in their struggles.

Addiction isn't just a choice; it's a complex interplay of emotional, physiological, and societal factors.

Bonds that Bind: The Circle of Dependence

The cycle of addiction is akin to a whirlpool. Once caught, the downward spiral intensifies. As dependence grows, so do the negative consequences. Job losses, broken relationships, and declining health are common markers on this treacherous path. With limited resources and societal stigmatization, the streets often become the last refuge. Fighting for necessities can exacerbate the cycle, making escaping back to normalcy even harder.

Addiction doesn't merely imprison the individual; it ensnares everyone around them. My niece lost everything, from her job to her relationships and the trust of everyone who loved her. She found herself going from friend to friend, sleeping on their sofas. She ended up ruining those friendships, too.

Most heartbreakingly, she lost custody of her firstborn due to her drug abuse. A pain unimaginable to most. However, this loss was a gift, a saving grace for my niece. This loss became the crucible of her transformation. Though the journey was steeped in pain, it culminated in hope. While it may have seemed "too late" in the eyes of some, she turned her life around. We're thankful that her child remains within our family, a beacon of faith, hope, love, and a reminder of what's at stake.

Hope Beyond the Horizon

It's not all gloom and despair. Stories of addiction may be prevalent, but so are tales of redemption, resilience, and rebirth. For every narrative of descent, there's one of ascent. Countless organizations, communities, and individuals are dedicated to helping those battling addiction. Efforts from rehab centers to community outreach programs are in full swing to pull those trapped and willing to participate out of the cycle. My niece's journey is a testament to that resilience. It's about more than just sobriety; it's about rebuilding lives and mending broken spirits.

Furthermore, society's growing understanding of addiction as a health issue rather than a moral failing is paving the way for more compassionate and effective interventions. The emphasis now is on sobriety and holistic wellbeing – addressing the root causes and providing the tools and resources for sustainable recovery.

So, the lingering question is: What can you do?

Your Role in the Larger Tapestry

Breaking the chain of addiction requires collective effort. From awareness to action, every gesture counts.

You can:

Educate and Advocate: Familiarize yourself with addiction's complexities. This isn't just about drugs or alcohol; it's about understanding the underlying factors – trauma, mental health, societal pressures, and more. [My niece has faced challenges with anxiety due to past childhood experiences. She's always yearned for acceptance, prefers company over solitude, and often aligns herself with group thinking.] Although each person is unique, these behaviors may indicate underlying issues that could be risk factors for addiction. Always approach any situation with empathy and understanding.

Volunteer: Lend a hand at local shelters, rehab centers, or community outreach programs. Your time makes a difference.

Donate: Every penny can help fuel the mission of organizations working towards breaking the cycle. Whether it's money, food, clothes, or books, your contribution can bring warmth to someone's day.

Listen: There are moments when we all need someone to listen to us. To be heard. We should engage in meaningful conversations, show empathy, and always remember that judging others can be easy, but it can also isolate those fighting their own battles. We've not walked in their shoes and should remember that Scripture teaches us to avoid being judgmental and to practice forgiveness.

To a Tomorrow Without Chains

The journey from the shackles of addiction to the light of hope is challenging but not impossible. My niece is the perfect example. Today, she is happily married with a two-year-old child and has a great relationship with her firstborn. It's a daily journey, but she understands that with a clear mind and focused thoughts. We will always be grateful for having her back, healthy, happy, and productive.

As we strive to understand, support, and uplift, we inch closer to a world where stories of addiction are fewer, and tales of recovery are the norm.

Are you ready to play a part in creating a brighter tomorrow? Start today, make a difference, and be the beacon of hope in someone's story.

Thea Nelson ~ *Amid life's storms, my unwavering trust in God has been my anchor. He steered my family through this crisis, strengthening my hope, deepening my faith, and growing my love for Him.*

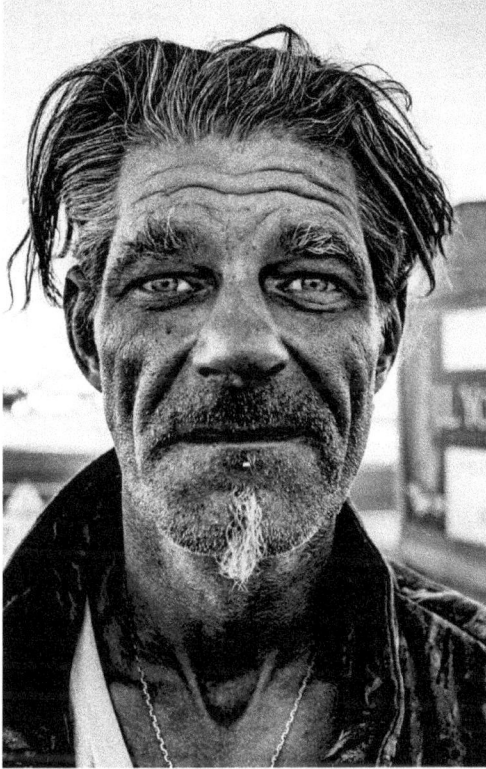

Dignity No Matter What: Collector Edition 2023
Renato Rampolla

Robert

"Times have been better," he said as he looked over at his wife, Molly, and their black lab, along with all of their belongings stacked over six feet high in a shopping cart alongside the road.

They had just been evicted after Molly's illness, which resulted in the loss of half of their income. They were on their way to Atlanta, where they heard social service agencies were more plentiful.

It's Not Where You Live But Why

By Judge Santiago Burdon
San Jose, Costa Rica

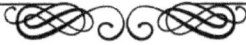

*I'm the only friend I've got
and I'm not sure he's one I can trust.*

Judge Santiago Burdon

I frequent dark alleys, empty railroad yards, abandoned buildings, park benches, and, at times, local jails. My only companion is my reflection in storefront windows when I pass. Occasionally, it surprises me when I show up at the duck pond at the local park. Pigeons no longer gather around me for breadcrumbs or stale popcorn. Those rats with wings finally realized I had nothing to offer and now ignored me, which worked out just dandy. I despise those filthy, lazy, annoying birds.

Fortunately, I've struck up a close friendship with the two very large and aggressive geese that have crowned themselves Emperor and Empress of the Park Pond. I named the pair Napoleon and Josephine. They no longer run at me, honking loudly, attacking me by biting my legs.

A short time back, there was a stray dog that took to me. The reason he befriended me, I believe, was because he saw me as an easy mark, which I probably am. I must've picked a couple of hundred ticks off of his body. He was welcomed company for the few weeks we spent together as pals. I named him Boondocks for some unknown reason. He would enthusiastically scamper up to me whenever I called for him. He looked to be a mix of Labrador and Shepherd. I knew him to be an affectionate and loving dog. I threw balls for him that he'd find near the tennis courts on the far side of the park.

He let me believe I taught him to retrieve when actually he taught me to throw the ball. He would sleep with his head on my chest and had an appetite like a grizzly bear. I never seemed to have enough food for the both of us. And I could see the disappointment in his pathetic brown eyes, staring at me, attempting to make me feel guilty.

The day finally arrived when he no longer returned when I called for him. His departure did cause me to become somewhat depressed. I even went to the Doggy Detention Center to investigate if maybe he'd been arrested, but I didn't find him there. I worried about his welfare, hoping he wasn't injured or worse.

Then, I spotted him in the park a month or so later. He looked clean, and his coffee-colored coat shimmered in the sunlight. His hair was brushed and no longer tangled and matted. He appeared to have gained some needed weight as well. He was accessorized with a bright red collar and a matching red leash complimenting his brown fur.

Daphne, a hooker I've known for a few years, was walking him. He acted as though he didn't know who I was, completely ignoring me. He pranced on by as though he was an AKC-registered purebred canine. I understood his reason for abandoning me. I didn't have any hard feelings about his decision. He traded up. He made the right move.

There's one stumbling block I can't seem to overcome: It's begging for spare change. I'm just no damn good at it. I don't have the talent for what it takes to be a successful panhandler. It's not because I'm too proud or embarrassed to beg for dimes and quarters. People don't seem to take me seriously.

Most folks try to avoid me by walking around me like I'm dog shit on the sidewalk. Others act as though I'm a con man trying to bilk them out of a quarter. My delivery doesn't seem to be convincing, or maybe I don't appear to be needy. Some go out of their way to humiliate me. They scream insults as they pass by.

"Get a job, you worthless bum."

"Piece of shit drug addict, alcoholic. I'm not gonna support your habit."

"The world would be a better place if you just killed yourself. "

You get the picture. There was a time when I took offense to jerks bad-mouthing me. Over time, I got used to it. I learned to ignore their derogatory comments, and instead, I thanked them for their suggestions. However, my comment seemed to infuriate some. Then I'd use the magic phrase, sure to defuse their anger. "God Bless You," I'd reply with a sincere expression. It worked most of the time, but occasionally there'd be a response of "Go screw yourself!" But it wasn't often.

There was a guy called Jingles, who I asked to teach me the "Ins and Outs" of the panhandling profession. He was a tall, lean fellow with a Southern accent. His sense of humor was always prevalent, and I'm not sure I ever saw him in any other mood. Most everyone looked up to Jingles. He had that kind of leadership quality about him. Also, he had a striking resemblance to Clint Eastwood and carried himself in the same manner. Jingles was a professional panhandler who never seemed to be unsuccessful.

I assumed the nickname Jingles was given to him because of the sound change made in his pocket. But that would be too obvious, making his moniker uninteresting without any real story behind it.

Someone mentioned he was once a Lieutenant in the Salvation Army. During the Thanksgiving and Christmas holiday seasons, he stood outside shopping malls or major department stores collecting donations from shoppers with a big red bucket. He'd ring a bell or shake a string of Jingle Bells. And that's how he got the name Jingles.

I was curious why he wasn't with the Salvation Army any longer. I asked around about his dishonorable discharge. The story's events changed depending on who was telling it. Basically, he had helped himself to a large sum of the donated cash. He skipped town, borrowing the Director's car and taking his nineteen-year-old daughter as well. They were arrested about a week or so later in Adams Friendship, Wisconsin.

Surprisingly, the Director refused to press charges. He didn't want his daughter subjected to the embarrassment of a trial. He also thought the publicity would hurt the local chapter of the Salvation Army. So Jingles ended up only doing three months in the county lockup.

I asked if I could partner with him the next day for some "on-the-job" training. He agreed, but with the condition that I didn't tell anyone, and he got twenty-five percent of my take.

He showed up at my camp around 7:30 in the morning, which I thought was early to begin training in "The Art of Panhandling." As we began to leave, he stopped me with his hand pushing against my chest. He started in on me about my clothes.

Reprimanding me, he said, "You're dressed too damn pretty."

"You got any other clothes that don't make you look like a used-car salesman? Maybe a dirty or torn shirt and a pair of pants don't fit good? That maybe is a little too big for ya?" He asked in a disgusted tone.

"Damn, Jingles, if I knew we had to have uniforms, I would have been prepared, but you never mentioned it."

"Doesn't it make sense to you that people aren't gonna give money to a guy wearing Docker slacks and a shirt from Old Navy? And Jesus Christ, look at your shoes, polished with matching shoelaces. What the hell kinda shoes are those?"

"Allen Edmonds," I confessed.

"So you're homeless, but you get dressed up every day to hang in the park? You think someone is gonna come around and offer you a job? For God's sake, you're wearing socks. You're dressed much too fancy. You'll never be on the cover of Tramps & Bums Magazine." He hollered sarcastically.

"Hey, you didn't give me an employee handbook or instructions on what to wear. Is there anything else I should know?"

"Yes, there is. What's your disability? You know, a physical handicap."

"I'm deaf in my right ear, my vision is impaired, and I've been diagnosed with Bipolar Disorder."

"No! I mean a prop for the con, like a broken arm in a sling or a foot injury walking with crutches. People are more sympathetic when they see a homeless person with a disability. They feel better about giving."

Damn, I didn't know he'd be so hard on me.

"I'll get it right next time. So where are we headed, Professor?"

"We're going to the Winn-Dixie parking lot. It's Saturday morning, and most housewives do their weekly food shopping on Saturday. Why would that statement be true, Mr. Ivy League?"

"Because most husbands get paid on Fridays. The wives want to buy groceries before their husband has a chance to blow the money at the track or the casino. Who knows? He might spend it on new tires for his car, or maybe he buys new fishing gear, or maybe…," Jingles interrupts.

"Okay, okay, Mr. Quiz Show contestant, you get a Gold Star. You like to hear yourself talk, don't cha?"

"Just answering your question, boss."

The Winn-Dixie parking lot was close to full of minivans and station wagons. The area bustled with the activity of suburban housewives heading to the entrance with kids in tow and others exiting with shopping carts full of next week's menu items.

"Now you can pick out the ones with a lot of groceries and ask if they need help. Most of the time, it involves a generous tip and maybe a piece of fruit. I don't go in for that kind of stuff; it's too much like work."

"What if you're asked to help? Do you say no?"

"Are you retarded or just playing dumb? You smile and give an enthusiastic 'Yes.' If they ask, there's surely a generous tip involved."

"Okay, got it."

The day became progressively better and more profitable now that I had been tutored on how to start an introduction.

The phrase, "Do you have any spare change?" is much too direct and crass, lacking a show of manners. Jingles created what he called the "pitch."

"Excuse me, can you help me with a small amount of loose change, please?" Said with a half grin, in a quiet voice as if you're embarrassed. It's much more polite.

I worked the housewives like a vacuum cleaner salesman and loaded quite a bit of groceries into vehicles. And just like Jingles said, I was raking in cash. My pocket was full and somewhat heavy from the change. I also received my share of apples, peaches, and bananas.

I was preparing to take a break and enjoy an orange when Jingles walked up on me from behind with the stealth of a Ninja.

"So how ya doin' rookie? Have you had a good day?"

"Ya. I think I did pretty well for my first time as a professional panhandler. Both of my pockets are filled with change. I haven't had time to count it."

"We can do that back at camp. Let's get to heading home. What do ya say?"

He called it home. After the six years I've lived on the streets, I have never referred to it as home. We walked back to camp without sharing much conversation. The sun displayed its last glint of light, painting the sky and the clouds with pink and red colors.

I gathered branches and pieces of wood from a pallet to make a fire. Jingles relaxed on the beach lounge chair I found in the garbage near the pool at the park. I replaced the missing straps with pieces of rope. The fire quickly transformed into a small blaze of dancing flames.

"This is a very comfortable piece of real estate you got here."

"Ya, I feel safe here. Although, every once in a while, some squatters try to claim my spot. But when I show back up with some members of the 'Street Legion,'* it results in a nonviolent eviction. I had one of those tents the church gave out last Christmas, but somebody ripped me off."

"Ya, they stole mine too, the bastards. So you got anything to drink around this place?"

"All I've got are four warm beers. My deluxe refrigerator broke down last week. I've been meaning to get it repaired." I answered.

"You're a real funny guy. Ever think about being a comedian?" He suggested in a sarcastic tone.

"Ya, when I was younger. I told my Old Man that's what I wanted to be. He said not to tell anyone I wanted to be a comedian because everybody would laugh at me."

"Now you're really cracking me up." He laughed while grabbing the beer I handed him.

"Let's take a look at how I did on my first day as a panhandler." I pulled the change from my pockets along with a few dollar bills.

"You got paper money as a tip?"

"Ya, I was surprised."

I earned $42.75 for my day's work. I counted out $10.50 and gave it to Jingles. He reached over and punched me in my right arm.

"Thanks for the payment. Hope you learned something. Hey, if you don't mind me asking, tell me how you ended up on the streets. I mean, you're intelligent, good-natured, not an addict or touched in the head, You know, crazy. And you're almost as good-looking as I am. Unless you're a wanted criminal on the run. In that case, no need to say anything. So come on, man, give me the skinny."

"First off, you're right. I'm not an addict, although I was in the past. But one morning, I woke up and just decided to give it up. It wasn't fun anymore. So I got clean. The criminal part—I'm not wanted or on the run as far as I know. However, some may consider me a criminal. I've never physically harmed anyone, nor did I burglarize or steal anything; I'm just not wired that way. You know, to be a thief. I worked as a drug runner for a Mexican Cartel a long time ago. Most people consider that to be a criminal act. So I guess I'm a criminal."

"It's bullocky, but unfortunately, it's true. So how did you end up here?"

"I've often thought about the event that has contributed to my present residency in the streets. It definitely didn't involve very much investigation. Ya see I'm an emotional cripple, a coward, unable to face the consequences of my decision. The guilt, the grief, and the heartbreak were too much to bear."

"Listen, I don't want you to talk about anything that's gonna cause you misery or make you come undone."

"I need to come clean with myself. And I want you to know I'm not the kind to openly discuss the circumstances surrounding my structured devastation. It's been years since I've faced my demon. I suppose now is as good a time as any."

Jingles got up to throw a couple more pieces of wood on the fire, then grabbed another beer out of the bag.

"Okay, if I have another beer?"

"Sure."

"Go ahead with your story. Sorry for the interruption."

"When my daughter was only 16, she was traveling from Portland along with a friend to visit me in Austin. While her friend was driving on a straight section of smooth highway, she ran off the road, crashing into a deep ravine.

My daughter was ejected while sleeping in the back. Her head violently slammed into the hard asphalt highway surface. The impact resulted in severely fracturing her skull. She sustained irreversible brain damage as well as other significant injuries. After CT Scans and other tests, the Neurologist explained his diagnosis. The list of injuries was extensive and took a long while for him to finish. He was concerned with my feelings, inquiring about my emotional condition after each injury was addressed.

"I wish I had better news for you concerning her head injury. Should I wait until your wife is available to give my diagnosis? When will she be available?"

"Please don't judge her absence as being unconcerned. She has stood by McKenzie's side for the past 48 hours. She's both physically exhausted and emotionally spent. I believe it would be a wise choice to let me give her the prognosis," I suggested.

He shook his head in agreement. Then he proceeded to tell me some of the most devastating information I've been subjected to in my entire life. He explained the best-case scenario with a compassionate tone and somber expression. McKenzie's quality of life, even if she fully recovered from the other injuries, would be bleak at best. He apologized for delivering such horrible news. We shook hands, and I thanked him for his efforts. I couldn't hold back my tears.

"Santiago, this is tearing me up inside."

McKenzie died the next day during her sixth episode of seizures, causing a massive heart attack. The medical staff worked to keep her alive. Then, I made the decision for them to quit with their efforts to resuscitate McKenzie without first consulting my former wife.

"Stop, that's enough. Let her go! Please just stop and let her go," I hollered in a commanding tone.

I stood at her bedside and watched my daughter die. I alone was determined to let her pass. It was my decision. It was the most agonizing and painful decision I've ever made in my entire life. I wouldn't want any parent to experience that kind of living Hell. There were those who harbored an animosity toward me, including my family, relatives, and close friends. It took a tremendous toll on me."

"That's a rough road to travel. I'm sure it felt like a punch to your gut. I'm sorry, man."

"Thanks, Jingles. I didn't respond well to her loss. I couldn't find the will or desire to answer the bell for the next round. So I just knuckled under. The grief became overwhelming, along with the guilt of being the one who gave the order to let her die. And the anger expressed by everyone I knew. It seemed as though the entire world blamed me.

I want you to know I blame no one but myself for my present situation. I accept that I'm less than half the man I once was. Now I'm looked at as an old guttersnipe, a scourge, a scab on the face of God. I've learned to swallow the taste of shame."

"Stop punishing yourself. Quit beating yourself up. I'm sure you did the right thing. Wanna know the way I see it?"

"Ya, tell me."

"It'd be a lot easier to feel sorry for yourself in the other world than it is here. Why sentence yourself to life on the streets? You could get outta here if you really wanted to. You've got all the skills and tools to make it."

"Easier said than done. But thanks for your advice. I'll take it into consideration."

There was the sound of leaves rustling along with underbrush coming toward the camp.

"Who's out there?" Jingles hollered.

"You better answer us. We can hear you out there," I added.

Appearing through the tall weeds surrounding the camp was a familiar face I hadn't seen in what seemed like years.

"I can't believe it. Boondocks, what are you doing back here?

"Out slumming, are ya?"

He ran to me and immediately began to dance around in a jerky fashion.

"Be careful, Santi, that dog is acting like it might be possessed. He could have rabies or something. Is it your dog?"

"He was mine, or maybe I was his once. He got a better offer and left without as much as a goodbye."

"See, you've got somebody. He found his way back home."

"You're right. Welcome home, Boondocks. Welcome home."

At 70 years old, the opportunities to support myself are scarce, although, sometimes, I get temporary assistance from a relative or fan of my books. It eventually comes to an end, finding myself back in my familiar home on the streets.

*Street Legion: Many large homeless areas have a group of protectors, somewhat like a police force, that settles disputes and acts of violence. They aren't elected but self-appointed, Usually made up of people with strong religious beliefs.

Judge Santiago Burdon ~ *Boondocks, thanks for your friendship.*

Being Homeless

By Russ Johns
Portland, Oregon, and Seattle, Washington

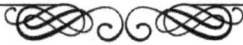

Kindness is cool and Smiles are free.

Russ Johns

Suicide, Hopeless, and Homeless

*W*e grow up thinking things are a certain way. We imagine what our life might look like and how we would like it to play out. Our ideas evolve from our experiences, the experiences of others, and our imagination.

"Experiments Become Experience"

However, life often has other plans for us. The only thing I wanted to be was a rock star!

I was on the path and played music professionally for several years, until life took a *hard* and abrupt turn in 1987 when I fell three stories from a billboard.

Launching from a Ladder… I came crashing down.

Did I mention *hard?*

Luckily, a young boy with his mother across the street saw me fall, and he said to his mom, "Geeze… That man just jumped from the billboard."

I was still conscious and looked up. Then I looked at my body and thought, "This is not good."

After getting admitted into the ICU by luck or by grace, the wonderful doctors patched me up.

I continued to find the help I needed to persist through two solid years of rehab, reconstruction, and medical challenges.

I survived.

Eventually, the company I worked for hired me back as their safety director because I knew what gravity was all about.

I wrote fall-protection programs and safety manuals and became an instructor in First Aid and CPR, defensive driving, crane safety, and another safety program. I then taught the individuals in the organization the skills needed for their job.

I soon ascended to another rung of the ladder. I became the IT Director, learning technology and project management to develop solutions and software for the corporate office.

So here I was, climbing the corporate ladder. I made it up to the corporate office, becoming the Director of Communications.

Big title, big budget, lots of pressure, limited sleep, and anti-depressants. The life I created was slowly killing me. Travel, corporate life, and then coming home to be Farmer Johns had a price.

By then, I had two boys of my own and was living in paradise on 30 acres on the Olympic Peninsula in Washington.

We had a hobby farm with llamas, cows, horses, chickens, and pigs. We were raising a family. We grew lavender, created a farmers market, and lived the dream.

It looked wonderful from the outside, but I was miserable and exhausted mentally, emotionally, and spiritually. I spent more time commuting and traveling than with my family until I was launched from that ladder of "Mergers and Acquisitions."

There was no little boy across the street to save me this time. No ICU, no nurse, no doctor to patch me up.

The company was sold, and the new management no longer needed my services. I was tossed into the corporate orphanage. I had given fifteen years of hard work to the company, but that was no relief from the pain I felt.

The dream became a nightmare, and then it changed even further. Not only had I just lost my 15-year career, my wife then asked me for a divorce.

I looked at the situation and said to myself, "This is not good."

I lost the farm and judged myself harshly. I'd worked hard for a life that was an illusion, the life I thought I wanted. I lost my family, I lost my job, and I was homeless. I was suicidal and was ready to check out.

And then something snapped.

I realized no one is responsible but me.

I committed to taking care of the boys and working on myself.

I had to turn inward. I worked on my health, what they call "self-care" today. I took some time off. I needed to figure some things out for myself.

"Invisible Homeless"

With no place to go, no job, no home, and no options, I became one of the "Invisible Homeless."

I was lost and needed to find some meaning to the chaos in my life, to redefine my life.

How did I do this? I organized everything, stripping my life down to the necessities. I started to camp out by couch-surfing with friends and living in my car. Everything I owned fit into three equipment bags. I bought a tent, put my mountain bike on the rack, and began to enjoy the real camping lifestyle.

I could get on the road and go camping for months. I traveled to Mexico with my oldest son and a few friends, and I built a church. I got back into music and biking. Slowly, I worked my way out of the darkness and despair.

I got baptized in the Pacific Ocean while building that church, hoping that whatever happened was meant to be.

I asked myself "What can I accomplish now?" I had no answers except for what was before me that day.

But I started to feel free.

One trip was a wonderful vacation with the boys. We went to Washington, Idaho, Montana, Yellowstone, Wyoming, Arizona, California, Oregon and back to Washington. It was an epic trip that all of us would remember.

I spent time on the road traveling to see my parents' relatives, journaling to discover what I needed to do next.

The idea that kindness is cool and smiles are free unfolded before me.

I was learning to be patient with myself, to be open to grace and gratitude, and to always be kind.

All kinds of thoughts appear when you go down the road with nothing except the voices in your head. But slowly, things got quiet inside my head.

I had adventures, tragedies, and many sleepless nights wondering what I was here for. What would I do next? What could I accomplish and how could I help?

I wanted to *help more people help more people.*

After over a year of couch-surfing, camping, traveling, journaling, and having some candid conversations with myself, helping people help people became my mission in life. I adopted a new sense of seeing. I felt alive for the first time in a long time. New opportunities were opening, and the stressful demands of life were falling away.

I felt free of the expectations that I once had. I begin to create something fresh and start something attractive to me.

I felt I needed to create in a way that I could help more people help more people, so I got a job as an inside salesperson for technology, and I rented a small apartment near my work to avoid the commute.

I couldn't imagine what life had planned for me when I first started falling from ladders, but now I see. I became victorious in my own life, continuing to camp, sleeping in my car when I wanted, and taking adventures with my boys.

Today, *kindness is cool, and smiles are free* is the motto I live by, and I share it freely with others as I continue to traverse this life.

Russ Johns ~ *I have to thank all the friends and family who helped me find a way to return from being last and homeless to having the confidence to return to a life worth living.*

No Shame in Your Game

By John Dunia
USA

It would be difficult to imagine a more ominous circumstance than being on the brink of homelessness. For those who've never faced this nightmare, it would be even more difficult to imagine the paralyzing amount of fear and anxiety that would immediately grip any person who has been given this devastating news.

Another emotion that frequently accompanies fear and anxiety is shame. All three of these emotions are devastating on their own; however, of these three, shame can be one of the most difficult to navigate because it is often minimized and misunderstood.

> *Shame is one of the most devastating emotions*
> *humans can possibly experience and*
> *it only gets stronger by feeding on itself.*

Becoming homeless makes every task seem more grueling and complicated. Even asking someone for help suddenly feels like a shameful deed. "What will others think about me?" or "I'm sure they will judge me and wonder what I did to put myself in this position."

These kinds of thoughts are typically brought on by shame. And the more we allow ourselves to dwell on negative thoughts like these, the quicker we are robbed of our ability and our will to take action to remedy our current condition. And the last thing anyone in this predicament needs is a declining sense of self or purpose.

Unfortunately, there is very little access to emotional well-being for those who are homeless. Many communities have organizations dedicated to helping people get back on their feet. Thankfully, they have been a Godsend to many. However, effective emotional help is often provided by therapists or other mental health experts, putting it out of reach for low-income individuals and families.

As the Shame Doctor, I'd like to share some helpful tips, practical advice, and valuable techniques that will help you overcome the shame you may be facing and empower you to build self-esteem as you strive to get back on your feet.

The first step is to truly understand what shame is. What exactly is shame, and how do we experience it? How does it impact our lives and occasionally control our decisions and choices? And why is it so easily confused with guilt?

Shame is the culmination of all the negative things we've come to believe about ourselves. Shame also tries to convince us that we truly are all those terrible things people have said we are and that we can't do anything to change or fix it. Believing there is no way of changing or fixing those traits is, without a doubt, the most devasting impact shame has on us.

We are not born with shame, but many of us experience it at an early age. It starts with the words of others and mainly from those we've come to love and trust. As infants, we naturally learn to trust others and tend to believe what they tell us is true. If their words express something terrible about us, we will likely believe it and be very disappointed in ourselves, which is how we begin to experience the feeling of shame.

When these interactions occur often, it becomes a ripe environment for shame to grow and strengthen. Eventually, many of us will fall into the trap of accepting that this is precisely who we are as if it were a fact. Perceiving it as a fact convinces us that we can do nothing to change it and that we will forever be this way.

Shame is often confused with the word guilt.

"You must be feeling all kinds of guilt and shame" is how it's frequently used in a sentence. But have you ever wondered what their differences are? When asked to define the word shame, many people will often use guilt in their definition. While there are similarities, they also have two very distinct meanings, and the best way to understand their differences is to compare and contrast them in identical situations.

Before continuing to read, try thinking about some differences yourself. How do you believe they differ? What makes you feel guilt or shame? After reading the explanations below, this brief mental exercise may help you better understand their differences.

Let's say someone makes me angry, and I yell at them harshly and excessively. Afterward, I realized my response was out of line and felt bad about how I reacted. When we make a mistake or a bad choice and feel poorly about it, that is the feeling of guilt. It's the acknowledgment and acceptance of our actions. Sometimes, the feelings are so strong they cause emotional stress as well as physical discomfort or pain.

If I were to yell at that same person and experience shame, it would tell me I made that mistake because something is wrong with me. I'm just that way, and nothing can be done to fix it because that's who I am.

In many ways, guilt acts as a moral compass. The emotional and physical discomfort we felt during our last incident can help us remember not to make a similar decision in the future. Shame, on the other hand, has virtually no redeeming qualities. It wants us to believe that we had no choice but to make that mistake because we don't have the ability to make the right choice.

The reason for the confusion with guilt is that we experience the same mental and physical symptoms with both of these emotions. But guilt can be dealt with by a willingness to change our behavior. Shame typically requires under-standing, self-compassion, and healing before making any change.

Another way to understand how shame plays a role in your life is to think of it as a little devil on your shoulder urging you to make the wrong choice, yet there is no angel on your other shoulder in your defense.

Shame stacks the deck against you.

It often feels like it's a force outside our body, similar to an evil spirit enticing you. Unfortunately, you created that demon. Even though all those horrible things you learned to believe about yourself were told to you by others, your belief and acceptance of those lies created that devious monster who is keen on giving you the wrong advice.

The first step toward defeating it is recognizing it when it shows up in your life, those moments when you feel ashamed. Identifying it will help you learn to correct it. When you catch yourself feeling that way, be thankful and compliment yourself. Praising yourself may feel odd, but you've taken a huge step in your healing journey.

Typically, our reaction is to feel bad about ourselves for feeling bad about ourselves. But that was likely how we learned to cope with those feelings. It's time to break that habit and create a new way to react. Complimenting yourself is the opposite behavior that shame wants you to exude and a good step toward creating a new and positive reaction.

The next step to making that change is to forgive yourself. Forgive yourself for ever thinking you were those terrible things you believed about yourself.

Forgiveness plays a huge role in our emotional healing. Unfortunately, many of us thought that forgiveness should apply to others and not ourselves. Self-forgiveness almost feels selfish or undeserved; forgiving someone else is so much easier.

I know how difficult self-forgiveness can be because I struggled with it, too. One of the most shame-induced events happened to me as a young teenager, and it continued to haunt me for decades until I understood why I needed to forgive myself.

I grew up in a religious organization, and I revered its founder. He was charismatic, and I embraced every word he spoke. Around the age of ten, I remember him saying that God told him every word he should speak, and I eventually convinced myself that was true.

When I was fourteen, he accused me of something that I did not do. Not only did he rebuke me harshly, but it was in front of all my male classmates, which added to my embarrassment.

Unfortunately, while he was attacking and condemning me, I told myself, "I must have done something wrong," because God is telling him what to say, and God is never wrong. During his tirade, I convinced myself that I was wrong, and it was made worse by the fact that I had no idea what I did to raise his ire that much. The confusion added to my shame, and I felt incompetent, embarrassed, and unworthy.

Thankfully, decades later, I realized that the problem wasn't those harsh words he said to me; it was that I BELIEVED the lies he told me. I needed to forgive myself for ever believing those lies, even though, at that time, I believed that was my only choice. Forgiving myself was the catalyst I needed to change the way I thought about myself, and that allowed the emotional healing to begin.

One of the struggles with emotional healing is knowing when it occurs. When a physical wound heals, we often see the evidence. The cut scabs over, and eventually, the skin grows back, a sore muscle feels better, or other signs that signify the injury is being restored or cured.

Proof of emotional healing is more difficult to detect mainly because it transpires psychologically, and the results are invisible or intangible. That lack of solid proof often hinders us from believing any healing is occurring. Forgiving ourselves is an act of faith, allowing us to change the way we think about ourselves, which is how we heal most of our emotional wounds.

Sometimes, we may struggle to maintain that self-belief, but if you find yourself in that dilemma, just continue to forgive yourself for having those doubts. Questioning ourselves can be akin to reopening those old wounds and undoing some or all of the prior progress.

Since each of us has a unique upbringing, our emotional healing journeys will also be unique.

We may learn from others' experiences, but our paths will differ. That also means there is no "silver bullet" or one singular piece of advice that works for everyone. Self-forgiveness, however, is the one thing that can help all of us on our emotional healing journey.

The right therapist can have a tremendous impact on your emotional health, but it's not always a viable option for many. Thankfully, there are other resources available. A library can be a valuable place for help, and simply talking to caring friends is another way of easing the burden we often hold inside ourselves. Also, there are online groups that offer help free of charge.

If you decide to join a group, please use caution. They may not have been properly trained or may use ineffective techniques or ideas detrimental to the healing process. You are in charge of your healing journey, so if something doesn't feel right, you are not obligated to follow it.

Most importantly, never allow others to make you feel bad about who you are. Anyone who thinks that shaming you is helpful only demonstrates how little they know about emotional healing. Good intentions do not always translate into good results.

For those who want to show compassion and empathy towards people who are currently experiencing home-lessness and not make them feel ashamed, do your best to treat them with dignity. Consider them as you would a new colleague you're meeting for the first time. Look them in the eyes, be courteous, ask them their name, and if you can help, don't make it a big deal. You don't need recognition. You may find it difficult and feel uncomfortable at first, but the more you attempt it, the better you'll become. And the more people you'll help.

It is not an easy task for most people to unfetter themselves from the grasp that homelessness seems to encircle us with. Keeping a positive outlook as much as possible is a tremendous asset to your success. There are enough obstacles to overcome, and we don't need to cause more by feeling poorly about who we are. Thankfully, winning the battle against shame is also a skill you can carry with you for the rest of your life.

John Dunia ~ *Dr. Shannon Smith was my therapist and helped me learn how to overcome and help others on their journey as well.*

One Conversation Can Change a Life

By Blake Brouillette
Denver, Colorado, USA

If you want to change the world,
go home and love your family.

Mother Teresa of Calcutta

I was supposed to be the supportive one in the relationship. At least, this is what I believed the first few months of my missionary year with *Christ in the City*.

Though not free of pain or sorrow, I lived a blessed life compared to my homeless friends. However, in one interaction, this entire belief shattered and left me with an understanding of genuine friendship.

As a college student, I went on several mission trips to a nonprofit called *Christ in the City* in Denver, Colorado. It hooked me, and I kept returning. So, it was no surprise to my family and friends when I became a missionary for two years after graduating from college. Many organizations serve the poor and do excellent work, but the model of encounter at *Christ in the City* rocked my world.

Young adult missionaries volunteer for one or two years to live in the community and serve the chronically homeless on the streets. The homeless ministry consists of teams going on the same route for a full year, providing a consistent and constant presence to those they encounter.

The working model with the homeless is a ministry of presence and encounter. It can be described as "wasting time with people" in order to get to know them and address the root causes of rupture in their lives.

Rodger was one of the homeless men my team saw almost every day. With his boisterous personality, larger-than-life disposition, and booming voice, he was well loved by anyone he interacted with. The first time I met Rodger on a mission trip to *Christ in the City*, I could not believe "people like him" were on the streets (you can see my ignorance at this stage of my life).

Rodger is a great example to flip the script on who you meet on the streets. Every conversation was diving into a book of an intriguing life made for a novel. Rodger was a college football player, the former CEO of a grain trading business, and had two children my age. He was a world traveler, and one of our favorite conversations involved Rodger planning my future vacations based on his past trips and expeditions. Rodger did have his issues and willingly let us into the struggle and accompany him during his journey. As Rodger shared these deep and authentic aspects of his life, my convinced mentality of keeping my struggles from Rodger was almost sterile.

My personal aim in going to the streets was to stay constant. I would laugh, rejoice, and share in sadness, but not too much. If I let myself get too excited, I would inversely be similarly affected by sadness. The threshold for highs and lows is mysteriously connected, so I made sure to hang in the middle.

One day, in particular, hanging in the middle proved extremely difficult. I had both external and internal suffering, that was penetrating every thought and interaction. Yet, I put on my neutral mask, and our team started walking our route.

The gloomy day felt fitting, and I was pleased with the traffic noise from the busy street to distract me. Rodger usually could be found in the park, so I was surprised when he was sitting on a bench right at the beginning of our route. I was not ready to see Rodger that day. I had spent more time with Rodger than my other homeless friends, so I knew my mask needed to be securely fastened.

I approached Rodger and gave a cordial greeting. It did not pass the test. Rodger's face immediately sank into concern, and he asked me, "Blakey, what's wrong?" I knew I was in trouble because he had a fatherly tone I had not heard before. "Oh, nothing. Just a bit tired." I quickly snapped back to ensure the mask convinced him.

But Rodger persisted, "Blakey, what's wrong?" The genuine concern on his face was unmistakable. I only made one or two excuses before taking the mask off and flinging it aside. "Rodger, I'm really struggling right now."

I felt naked and exposed, like I failed in this moment. I had nothing to give. My head was down, and I felt defeated by the gaze of a man sitting on a park bench. I do not remember the following few moments of our conversation or what was shared between us. My memory goes to the end of the conversation, where Rodger looked at me with big brown eyes and with tears streaming down his cheeks.

He grabbed my head and pulled me close. "Blakey," he said with a cracked voice. "You go right into that Church." He pointed up the street toward the Catholic Cathedral. "You sit in those pews, and you tell your Father everything. Give it all to Him and let Him take care of you." The tears filled our eyes now, and we embraced in a long hug. The moment overflowed with Rodger's fatherhood, and his capacity of love directed towards me.

I walked away, not feeling defeated or exposed. The feeling was quite the contrary. I had been loved. By exposing myself and letting Rodger into my suffering, I opened my heart to the fatherly love he was capable of and showed so tenderly. The mask that had been "protecting" me for months was shattered and became oh-so brittle. The thing I looked to for safety was, in fact, a facade that prevented the deepening of friendship. Once it was removed, Rodger could show compassion and care towards me. He not only entered into my suffering but did so willingly.

Rodger's and my relationship would never be the same. I had called him my friend before, but a one-way relationship is not a friendship. Now, he was truly a friend. Friendship is a two way-street., supportive, loving, caring, and willing for the good of the other. Rodger willed my good as I willed his.

I continued to see Rodger regularly, and our relationship deepened. His greater trust in me could be seen, allowing me to challenge and call him higher in ways I could not before. At the same time, he challenged me, desiring healing and reconciliation in my life as a true father does.

One man and one moment changed my entire approach to my homeless ministry. Heck, my understanding of friendship changed. I learned to let people see me. It is risky but worth it. We are not made to fight our fights alone. I was convinced of this with my work on the streets, and it continues to ring true in my life and those I encounter.

"Homelessness is not a problem to be fixed, but a person to encounter."

The mission of *Christ in the City* is rooted in this ministry of encountering and meeting the poor where they are. To accomplish this, the program brings in young adult volunteers to be formed and go to the streets for a year or two of their lives. The volunteers, or missionaries as we call them, live in community life where they live a life of simplicity and sacrifice to make the mission on the streets possible.

Each year, the program brings in hundreds of volunteers of all ages to serve the homeless alongside the missionaries. There is a desire in society to serve the poor, but so many do not know where to begin. This is where *Christ in the City* and the mission come into play. By switching the view of homelessness as a problem to be solved to a person to be encountered, every person in society has the opportunity to individually address poverty. Material goods are needed and a must, but we must never lose sight of the deeper desire for connection and relationship that the poor so desperately need.

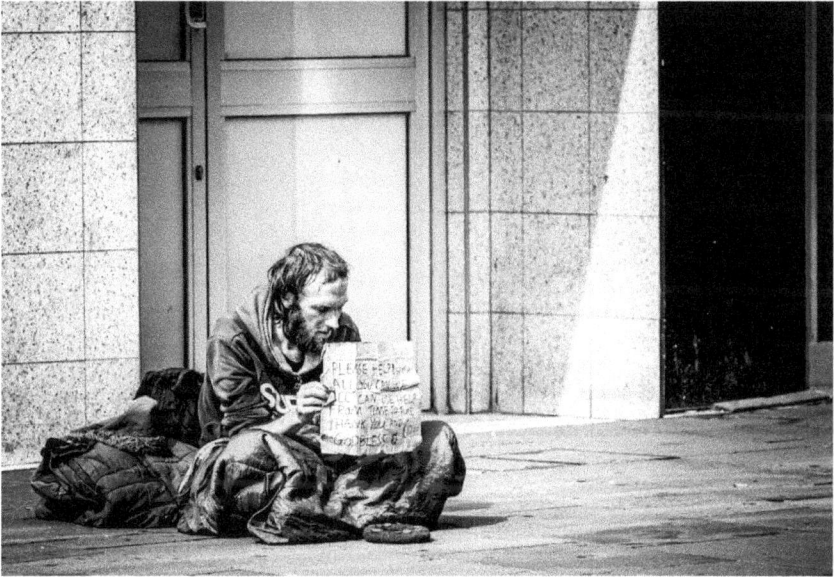

United Kingdom
Sarah Harvey, Photographer

I Can See Clearly Now

By Susan Rooks

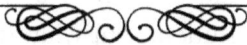

*A*dopted at birth, I was given great DNA from my creators and given a wonderful life with my (adoptive) parents. They later had another child – my mother's only pregnancy that gave me a younger brother – and we had a nice little family.

Solid middle class.

Nothing fancy, but always secure. There was always enough of what mattered, sometimes even a little bit more.

Loads of aunts, uncles, cousins. Only one grandfather, but he was an interesting man in his own way.

I grew up in the era that came right after WWII ended, and security, calmness, and sameness were prized. I had no idea how others lived; although we had a TV (one of the first color TVs) and two telephones, our lives were much smaller than is typical of today's world.

We were surrounded by those much like us – able to have a car (sometimes two) and a home, eat out occasionally, and even play golf at a local club.

We kids were really sheltered and very lucky, even though we didn't know it then.

I did the typical things that young women in my world did in the 1950s / '60s: I went to college (a two-secretarial school), worked for a couple of years as a secretary, met a guy, got engaged & married, and had two kids. Of course, I also stayed home after the birth of my first daughter as we did then; it was a rare woman who worked at that time when she had kids at home.

I had no real idea of how others lived outside our small circle, even though we ultimately hosted six international exchange students for up to a year. Of course, they came from different countries, so the stories they told didn't really impact us much. Even though we did learn a lot about life beyond our borders, our lives were quite different. Yes, the students' families clearly had enough to be able to send one of their kids to us as an exchange student, but what did that mean in terms of how they lived? We just assumed they had enough and never thought much about it.

So later, as I returned to work part-time (when my kids were old enough to be in school) and met more folks, I finally realized that not everyone had the same lifestyle as we did. We had a home that I figured would always be ours. My husband and I each had our own car. We had a motor home, basically an old bus with two areas for sleeping, a tiny bathroom, and a tiny kitchen/seating area.

In the summers, we traveled with our young kids up and down the East Coast, enjoying the different areas with their weather, towns, and people. We talked with others who lived there, learning a bit about their lives, but we usually spoke with those who seemed much like us.

We didn't see the "dark" side, the areas where the folks lived who didn't have much in the way of resources, ones that I had always just taken for granted.

A journey of a thousand miles starts with a single step.

My first exposure to even a tiny bit of the reality of harsh and often different ways others lived was in 2006 when a friend mentioned she was active in a local chapter of an organization called Habitat for Humanity (HFH), and she would be attending a meeting as a visitor in a couple of nights. Did I want to go with her?

Well, I had nothing else to do, so I said, "Sure!"

There were maybe a dozen visitors at that meeting, talking with the six or seven Board of Director (BOD) members about their next "build," something I knew nothing about. They explained a little of the background and process, including building homes for families who had no easy way to have a home of their own due to the costs.

Well, I realized that not everyone could afford to own a house, which is why so many rented apartments, but I hadn't realized that HFH even existed or that it filled that need around the world, one house at a time. All the labor came from volunteers, obviously alongside and supervised by professional builders, who also worked for free. The materials were donated by local businesses whose owners were interested in helping out.

And, no, the houses were NOT (and still are not) free to the homeowners. They also had to put in several hundred hours of work on it, either directly by themselves or with their friends or family. They ended up with a mortgage held by HFH, which was far smaller than the typical one. They also ended up with a brand new house, something they likely only dreamed of, not daring to believe it could really happen.

I loved everything about this organization, and I attended several meetings, unknowingly occasionally talking with folks who not only couldn't afford to buy a house conventionally but who didn't even always have a secure place to live. I heard a few small comments about some living in tents, but I don't think I even believed that.

Of course, each family that won the "lottery" of the next build in their area had to prove they could actually pay the mortgage and all other associated living fees, so I am sure we never really even talked with those whose application indicated they wouldn't be able to.

I stayed with that HFH chapter for five years, four as BOD President, helping to build five new homes in five years, a record for that chapter (and many others)!

One of the best lessons I learned during those years was the importance of accurate information to achieve the organi-zation's goals, especially those that depended on local folks' help. We understood that many town folks did think HFH gave free homes, so we decided to invite them to our monthly meetings to hear what we discussed.

To listen and learn the truths about the reality of folks NOT getting *a free* house.

To talk with us after our meetings and understand more clearly what we were doing and how they could help. And why they should.

Due to those monthly meetings with townspeople, we had a far more robust response when we announced that we were looking for help to build a house for a family in their town than we would likely have otherwise.

What was even better for me were the lessons I learned about necessary and accurate information being given, the wider world I began to see more clearly, and my growing need to be part of something bigger than I was.

360° Nation: All that is done is done "for good."

Fast-forward to 2023, and as one of the 360° Nation columnists, I began to widen my scope to see what else I could do within this marvelous organization that Dennis Pitocco started back more than 10 years ago. I've been one of the columnists for several years, and I'm also a member of a couple of the groups, notably GoodWorks 360°, working to help nonprofits around the planet as best we can.

So back in August 2023, when Dennis posted the idea of the anthology concerning the homeless: Bingo! Straight to my head and heart it went! I finally had a mission, something to do that would be and was far bigger than I am or any one person is.

That post touched something deep inside me, and I commented that it sounded like an extremely worthy endeavor. He and Peggy Willms then responded with a wonderful email, asking if I'd be interested in helping with this new venture, editing/proofreading the stories they hoped to receive from those who had been homeless or knew others who had been. They were using a new term – "Unsheltered" – for those with no secure or permanent place to live.

Dennis and Peggy agreed that I could be a part of the small team that would be putting this together. We would be asking for stories from folks and organizations around the world – not just the US – seeking to show their lives that perhaps started out with great expectations and then lost their way. Or those who had been unsheltered at some point in their life but were able to find a way to change that narrative for themselves, showing the possibilities that others could learn from.

I can see clearly now.

Now, many months later, it's been so much more than I had anticipated!

Like so many who haven't had the struggles of losing a home or a job or any other of life's other basic necessities, I had no real idea about those who lived in tents, on the sidewalks, under the overpasses in towns and cities, or in sheltered group homes.

Like far too many have done, when I saw someone holding up a sign at a traffic light or at the corner of a business area asking for money, I turned away. I had NO idea what else to do.

If anyone had asked me, I likely would have said it was really too bad, but maybe they just didn't have what it takes to succeed. Maybe they did something wrong, and this was the result.

Maybe – they didn't deserve anything better.

Maybe – they chose to live this way.

Maybe – they (fill in the blank).

But by the third or fourth story I read (now up to about 30), I began to see how blind I'd been. Not meaning to blame the victim exactly, but still … blind.

Blind to the reality that "ugly" could happen to any one of us: We could lose our job.

Expenses for ordinary things – rent, electricity, food – could rise above our ability to pay.

We could use up our meager savings because we suddenly need a few more dollars than we earned last week, month, or year.

Sickness and medical costs could take what little we managed to save.

Family members who used to help us suddenly couldn't help themselves, let alone help us.

And the biggest lesson of all?

**No one is guaranteed immunity
from difficulties; no one.**

Were my eyes opened?

Was my heart involved?

Do I see things differently now, as I had with HFH?

Do I applaud those who struggled and managed to move forward towards a far better life?

Do I hope that others who haven't made it quite that far yet learn how to do it?

Yes. Yes. Yes.

And I hope that as you read the stories in this exceptional anthology, your eyes will also open wide.

Your heart will beat in a different rhythm.

You will be inspired to find ways to help those who so need and deserve what we can do for them.

Maybe you actually did understand the reason(s) so many were unsheltered/homeless, but if not …

Do you see this more clearly now?

I know I do.

Conclusion

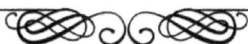

*A*s you close this book, remember that the stories within these pages are not just words—they are lives, experiences, and untapped potential. The unsheltered individuals you've met through these narratives are our neighbors, our fellow citizens, and, most important, human beings deserving of dignity and support. These accounts have given voice to those often silenced by society, illuminating the complex realities of homelessness and challenging long-held stereotypes. By reading their stories, you've taken the first step toward understanding and empathy. However, understanding alone is not enough; it must be the catalyst for action.

Now, it's your turn to become an agent of change. Whether through volunteering at local shelters, advocating for policy changes, or simply changing how you perceive and interact with those experiencing homelessness, you have the power to make a tangible difference. Challenge yourself to step beyond your comfort zone, engage with your community, and be a voice for those who have been marginalized. Share what you've learned, spark conversations, and inspire others to join this crucial movement.

By doing so, you'll improve lives and enrich your understanding of humanity and your place within it. Let this be the beginning of your journey to create a more compassionate, inclusive society—one where everyone has a voice, a home, and hope for the future. Together, we can rewrite the narrative of homelessness and build a world where dignity and opportunity are accessible to all.

Book Club Prompts

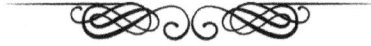

1. What is your overall takeaway after reading *Unsheltered: Voices from the Street?*

2. Has your opinion about those who are or have been unsheltered changed?

3. If you could pose a question to any of the contributing authors, what might you ask?

4. What is your community doing to address the needs and concerns with the unsheltered population?

5. What do you feel you can do to improve the epidemic of homelessness?

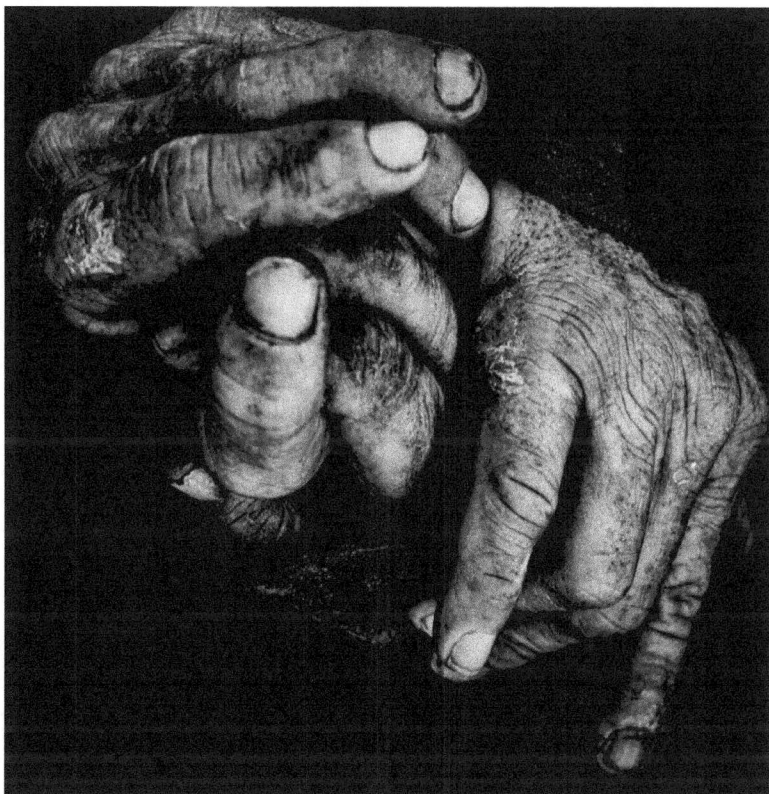

Dignity No Matter What: Collector Edition 2023
Renato Rampolla

Car Wash and Angel

"Together Always,"' Angel said as she and Car Wash held each other's hands.

"The name Angel I've heard before, but Car Wash?" I asked.

"They call me Car Wash 'cause I used to detail cars. Nice ones! Bentleys, Cadillacs, Lambos, and Benzes. People trusted me with their cars, and I detailed them better than anyone! Important people would wait until I had a time slot for them."

Meet The Co-Author,
Peggy Willms

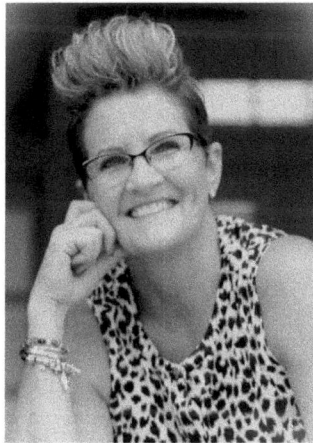

Peggy **Willms** has been a certified fitness trainer, sports performance nutritionist, and personal and executive health, wellness, and life coach for over thirty-five years. She is an entrepreneur, bestselling author, a featured contributor for BizCatalyst360, an international online magazine, hosts wellness retreats, and is host of The Coach Peggy Show.

She spent over twenty years in corporate wellness and has managed multi-million-dollar medical clinics. Her unique business and work-site wellness programs have earned her multiple awards. She has two sons and two grandsons. She loves all things beach and sunshine and lives in Florida with her better half.

https://linktr.ee/coachpeggy

Meet The Co-Author,
Dennis Pitocco

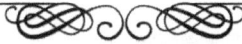

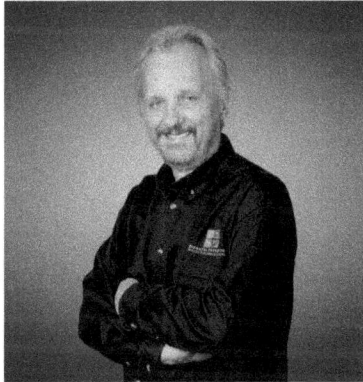

*D*ennis Pitocco is the founder and CEO of 360° Nation, a multifaceted media enterprise promoting global positivity. In collaboration with his wife Ali, who serves as Chief Inspiration Officer, Dennis oversees several successful ventures: BizCatalyst 360°– an award-winning global media platform; 360° Nation Studios – as producer of uplifting content and events; and GoodWorks 360°– a pro bono consulting service for nonprofit organizations worldwide.

For over a decade, Dennis and Ali have pursued a mission to illuminate the finest aspects of humanity and leverage their resources to effect daily positive change worldwide. Their operational philosophy emphasizes presence, compassionate service, and the allocation of time, talents, and resources for societal benefit rather than solely for profit. As a contributing author to multiple best-selling books, Dennis is committed to fostering transformational change and promoting holistic wellness.

Dennis and Ali strive to exemplify responsible stewardship while influencing and showcasing humanity's highest potential. Their work reflects a dedication to ethical business practices, community engagement, and the belief that media can be a powerful force for good in the world.

https://www.linktr.ee/dennispitocco

Meet David Berenbaum,
Foreword

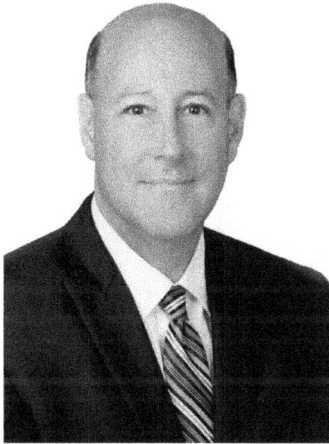

David Berenbaum is nationally known as a trusted voice for consumers and as a champion for a vibrant housing marketplace that celebrates the importance of fair and affordable housing, so that every neighborhood is a community of opportunity.

David serves as the Deputy Assistant Secretary for Housing Counseling at the United States Department of Housing & Urban Development and has held executive positions with the Homeownership Preservation Foundation, the National Community Reinvestment Coalition, the Equal Rights Center, the Fair Housing Council of Greater Washington, and Long Island Housing Services.

He is a frequent presenter at conferences across the nation – where he speaks from the heart and educates stakeholders to the importance of empowering consumers to make responsible choices to improve their housing, rally their credit and savings, understand their rights and responsibilities, and to avoid and/or recover from eviction, foreclosure, natural disasters, being unhoused or life's unanticipated hardships.

David has testified before Congress many times as a non-partisan subject matter expert, has served on many public and private sector advisory and social enterprise boards, has appeared as an expert on national news magazines and media shows, and has been regularly quoted by news sources across the country.

LinkedIn: https://www.linkedin.com/in/davidberenbaum/

Meet Renato Rampolla,
Photographer

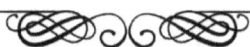

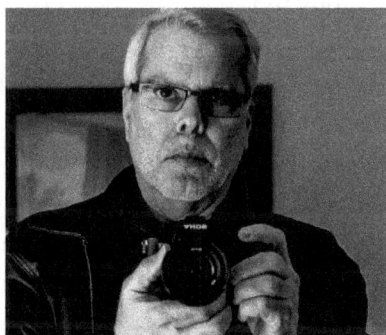

*R*enato Rampolla is an American lens-based artist. His interest is in exploring the fundamental aspects of humanity, particularly the intricate connections between individuals and societies, as well as our symbiotic relationship with the natural world. As an observer, artist and facilitator, he aims to foster a deeper understanding of what it truly means to be human.

He holds a B.A. in Social and Behavioral Sciences from the University of South Florida, which he obtained in 1983. Notably, Rampolla had the privilege of studying under the guidance of the sculptor, Jerry Meatyard, the brother of renowned photographer Ralph Eugene Meatyard, where he honed his skills in composition, color, and sculpting.

Rampolla has garnered recognition in various platforms. His work has been featured in Dek Unu Fine Photography Magazine, and his book, titled 'Dignity No Matter What: The Light Within,' which showcases intimate portraits of individuals living on the streets was juried into the 12th Annual Photobook Show on 2021 at the Davis Orton Gallery in Hudson, New York, and was also exhibited at the Griffin Museum of Photography in Winchester, MA.

Rampolla's work has been showcased in numerous gallery and museum exhibitions across the United States. His work has been featured in consecutive years (2022 and 2023) at the highly acclaimed Soho Photo Gallery National Competition in New York, NY. Other notable exhibitions that have featured his work include PhotoSpiva at the George A. Spiva Center for the Arts, National Exhibition in Joplin, MO, The SE Center for Photography in Greenville, SC, Praxis Photo Arts Center in Minneapolis, Minnesota, the ongoing online Lenscratch Fine Art photography exhibition, as well as exhibitions at The Mount Dora Center For The Arts, The Museum of Art and History in Maitland, FL, and The Museum of Art in Deland, FL.

Recognizing his artistic achievements, Rampolla has been honored with the Professional Development for Artists Grant on two occasions, from the esteemed Arts Council of Hillsborough County, FL..

mailto:renato@renatorampolla.com

Website: https://www.renatorampolla.com/

Meet Sarah Harvey, Photographer

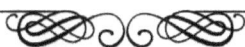

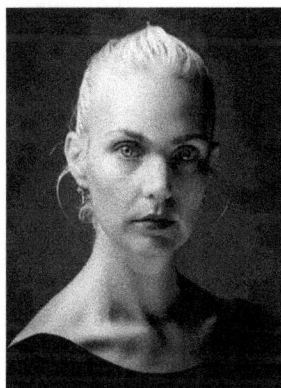

$\mathcal{S}$arah is a UK-based photographer specializing in light manipulation to create depth and mood in her subjects. Based in southern England, she leverages her contemporary fine art background to craft compelling compositions with organic narratives.

Sarah views her camera and lens as modern-day paintbrushes in our digital world. After earning her Master's degree from the prestigious Arts University Bournemouth in 2008, Sarah has cultivated a thriving career as both a studio and on-location photographer. Her talent has garnered international recognition, with short listings for the 'Black and White Photo Award' in both 2023 and 2024.

mailto: info@sarahharveyphotographer.com

Website: www.sarahharveyphotographer.com

Facebook: www.Facebook.com/sarahharveyphotographer
LinkedIn: https://www.linkedin.com/in/sarah-harvey-9aba051b4/
Instagram: www.instagram.com/sarahharveyphotographer

Meet Rocky Michaels, Singer/Songwriter

Unsheltered Anthem

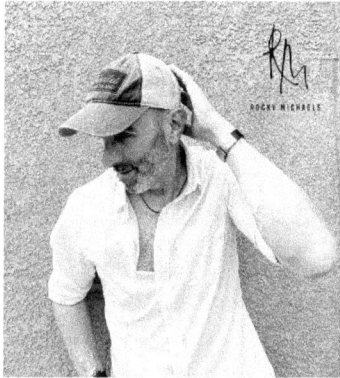

*R*ocky Michaels is a multi-award-winning American singer-songwriter/ recording artist. He has recorded three studio albums involving thirty-one officially released songs. Rocky began playing piano at age five and crafted his skills into songwriting throughout high school.

May 2024:

1. Rocky's tender ballad, "Better Man," climbed to #1 on the UK Talk Radio Hot 100 charts. (Official Music Video: https://www.youtube.com/watch?v=YC6gcvQStiM)

2. Nominated for "Male Artist of the Year Folk/Americana" by the Josie Music Awards held at the iconic Grand Ole Opry in Nashville, TN.

   Website: https://www.josiemusicawards.com/

November 2023: Rocky's song "An Uncomfortable Truth" was adopted as the anthem for a very special book endeavor dedicated to the homeless population around the world: Unsheltered: Voices from the Street
BizCatalyst: https://www.bizcatalyst360.com/an- uncomfortable-truth/

May 2023: Nominated for "Song of the Year Folk/ Americana" (Better Man) by the Josie Music Awards.

December 2020: Voted "Male Artist of the Year" by CFAB Music Realm Promotions.
Facebook: https://www.facebook.com/groups/cfabmusicrealm/permalink/511042436493927/

With several new songs currently in the pipeline, including a five-song EP scheduled for release by year's end, Rocky continues to tap into his life experiences to offer honest lyrics in storytelling that audiences have found to be both engaging and relatable.

"Rocky Michaels for me is that guy who stands out as one of my favorite music discoveries of 2020!!" (Jon Sexauer, Owner and CEO at The Grey Eagle Radio Show.)

An Uncomfortable Truth

(Music & Lyrics by Rocky Michaels)

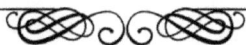

I see you walkin' down the street tryin' not to look at me
Does my appearance keep you away
I might be a tattered one but you don't know what I've got underneath as I fight
another day
A casualty I might be of a downsized economy
Or a suffering victim of disease
I might be a broken soul from a broken home just trying to piece things on my own
But you don't see the forest for the trees
Here, Here I Am
Will you even look me in the eye
Can you hear me talkin'
Or will you just keep walkin' by
Oh, well I am you and you are me and sometimes truth is hard to see
Everybody's got a story full of torn and weathered pages
Plots with twists and conflicts to unfold
You can judge me by my cover but if you took some time to read
A greater tale is waiting to be told
Well Here, Here I Am
Do you see me standing here at all
Can you hear me talkin'
Will you even answer to my call
Oh yeah, well I am you and you are me and sometimes truth is hard to see
There're eight billion souls of us now living

And eight billion reasons worth giving a little of ourselves
For years I kept praying and hoping
But my dreams they all left me long ago
I'm not bad but I'm not good at coping anymore
I guess I just wanted you to know
Well Here, Here I Am
Will somebody please make some time for me
Cause I fear you're missin'
More to my story than you see
Oh, well I am you and you are me though it might be uncomfortable to see
Na-na na na-na-na-na Na-na na
Na-na na na-na-na-na Na-yeah (I'm somebody too)
Na-na na na-na-na-na Na-na na (Whoo − hoo yeah)
Na-na na na-na-na-na Na-yeah (I am you and you are me, hey)
Na-na na na-na-na-na Na-na na (Yeah yeah, yeah yeah yeah)
Na-na na na-na-na-na Na-yeah (Woo - hoo)
Na-na na na-na-na-na Na-na na

Meet Our Publishing Team

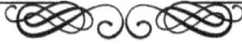

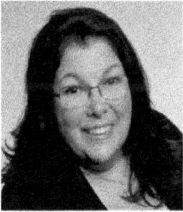

Teresa Velardi is the founder of Authentic Endeavors Publishing, a Multi Best-Selling Author, Speaker, Potter, Transformational Life Coach, and a Radio Host: Conversations That Make a Difference on DreamVisions7Radio.

https://linktr.ee/teresavelardi

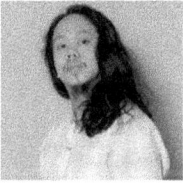

Aljon Inertia specializes in creating beautiful, one-of-a-kind illustrations for children's books. His goal and purpose are to bring his passion for illustration to children's books that speak to good morals and values while providing lessons to today's youth. His colorful illustrations engage the author's content, so the story comes alive in books worldwide. He also creates beautiful covers that bring the book title alive.

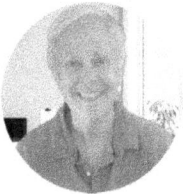

Susan Rooks is known as the "Grammar Goddess" and is an editor who specializes in helping authors of nonfiction and business-related documents. To date, she's edited more than 60 books from authors in several countries, often having to use their country's English grammar rules rather than the American ones she's most familiar with. She also helps with websites, résumés, blogs, and podcast transcriptions. Susan's only goal is to "help all authors look and sound as smart as they are."

LinkedIn: https://www.linkedin.com/in/susanrooks-the-grammar-goddess/

Meet The Contributing Authors

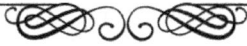

Mathew Broster is determined to help change this world but "I struggle myself and often feel insane, abnormal, and totally different to society." He believes his higher calling is to lead by example and be the voice for the voiceless before then handing them the mic. To him, humanity is in a state of disassociation, conditioning, fear, and ignorance, and he believes we are here to lead the way through love, leadership, connection, empowerment, and compassion.

mailto: mathewbroster15@gmail.com

Website: https://www.otsoof.com/

Facebook: https://www.facebook.com/profile.php?id=1000921682 68350&mibextid=ZbWKwL

Instagram: https://instagram.com/@offthestreetonourfeet

Noreen Braman is the daughter of laughter and chaos. "My life might sound like one trauma after another, and you might expect me to be depressed and sad. And yes, I have been. Yet, my nieces, nephews and grandchildren love me because (as they have said), I am always smiling. And that is what has sustained me, even when there was nothing to smile about."

mailto: info@njlaughter.com

Blake Brouillette is the Managing Director for *Christ in the City*, a missionary formation and homeless outreach program in Denver and Philadelphia. Blake was a missionary for two years, living in a community of volunteers and serving the homeless in Denver, Colorado. He is in his ninth year with *Christ in the City*.

mailto: blake@christinthecity.org

LinkedIn: https://www.linkedin.com/in/blake-brouillette-a64267161

Andi Buerger founded *Beulah's Place* (BP) and *Voices Against Trafficking* (VAT), two NPOs. They rescued 300+ at-risk homeless teens and successfully reintegrated them back into community. VAT is international. She is a survivor of child sex trafficking by family members. Her work with homeless youth and their experiences led to a conversation with this book's Co-Author, Dennis Pitocco, and is the basis for her chapter/article in this book.

mailto: andi@voicesagainsttrafficking.com

Facebook: www.facebook.com/voicesagainsttrafficking

LinkedIn: https://www.linkedin.com/in/andi-buerger-78372a238/

X: https://twitter.com/@VoicesAgainstT1

Instagram: https://instagram.com/@Voices_Against_Trafficking

YouTube: https://www.youtube.com/VoicesAgainstTrafficking

Judge Santiago Burdon's stories and poems have appeared in over three hundred magazines, literary journals, podcasts, and anthologies. Judge Santiago was recognized as an *International poet and author in Who's Who* of Emerging Writers 2020 and again in 2021. He has authored eight books published by three different distinguished presses and lives modestly in Costa Rica.

mailto: https://elchapo1225.sg@gmail.com

Facebook: https://www.facebook.com/9547albany

Joseph Carrabis has been everything from a long-haul trucker to a Chief Research Scientist and held patents covering mathematics, anthropology, neuroscience, and linguistics. He's the author of *The Augmented Man, Empty Sky, The Inheritors, Tales Told 'Round Celestial Campfires, The Shaman*, and the non-fiction neuroscience-based *That Th!nk You Do.*

mailto: joseph@nlb.pub

James Coleman is a devout lover of Christ, dedicated to the service of humanity either in business or just being in public. It's amazing the stories you can hear and learn if you just look at someone and smile and say, "Hello."

John Dunia has studied "shame" and how it frequently devastates the souls of people. However, the most important aspect is not shame itself, but how to heal from those devasting effects.
    mailto: johnsrep@gmail.com
    LinkedIn: https://www.linkedin.com/in/john-dunia-40400654/

Paul Fitzgibbons sold his Pilates studio five years ago, everything we had except two big backpacks full of clothes and necessities and began traveling the world. I am a writer writing as Jack Everly, traveling with my wife and daughter(s).
    mailto: pfitz905@gmail.com
    LinkedIn: http://linkedin.com/in/jack-everly-c-s-706283193

Julie Winkle Giulioni is an author, consultant, trainer, and speaker who helps organizations tap their only sustainable competitive advantage: talent. She is one of *One of Inc.* magazine's Top 100 speakers, and she's the co-author of the international bestseller, *Help Them Grow or Watch Them Go* and author of *Promotions Are So Yesterday: Redefine Career Development. Help Employees Thrive.*
    Website: http://www.juliewinklegiulioni.com/
    Facebook: https://www.facebook.com/JulieWinkleGiulioni.Author/
    LinkedIn: https://www.linkedin.com/in/juliewinklegiulioni/
    X: https://twitter.com/@Julie_WG
    YouTube: https://www.youtube.com/results?search_query=julie+winkle+giulioni

Earth O. Jallow is a small business owner, a mother, a doula, a professional West African Dancer, and a teacher. She is a 24-year radio/TV personality, writer, activist, voice-over artist, sign language interpreter, and forever student of life.
    mailto: peaceonearth07@gmail.com

Russ Johns is a speaker, creator, and author. His experience with trauma and resilience has significantly shaped his approach to life. After surviving a life-altering accident in 1987, he was inspired to give back to the community and speak about kindness and resiliency. His mission, "Help More People Help More People," reflects this commitment.

Website: https://russjohns.com/
Website: https://thepiratesyndicate.com/
Facebook: https://www.facebook.com/PirateBroadcast/
LinkedIn: https://www.linkedin.com/in/nextstepnext/
X: https://twitter.com/russjohnsdotcom
Instagram: https://www.instagram.com/russjohns/

Perry Knoppert is the founder of *The Octopus Movement*, transformed from homelessness to leading a global initiative, championing non-linear thinking for sustainable solutions. His life, mirroring mycelium's resilience, inspires a network of unconventional thinkers to address complex global challenges, showcased in the documentary *The Beauty Between Thoughts*.

mailto:info@theoctopusmovement.org
Facebook:https://www.facebook.com/groups/theoctopusmovement
LinkedIn: https://www.linkedin.com/in/perryknoppert/
LinkedIn: https://www.linkedin.com/company/the-octopus-movement/about/?viewAsMember=true
YouTube: https://www.youtube.com/channel/UCi9v1UaZgpvgZ_ynbrgtkGw

Cynthia Kosciuczyk is passionate about art and science. Writing and researching with a poetic style. Loves intelligent conversation and design. Believing optimism will triumph and hopes as an entrepreneur to make a difference in the world.

mailto: Cynthia@salonistasays.com
Website: www.salonistasays.com
Facebook: https://www.facebook.com/designertastes
LinkedIn:

https://www.linkedin.com/in/cynthia-kosciuczyk-bs-mba-4462127/
X: https://twitter.com/@salonistasays
Instagram: https://instagram.com/@salonistasez

Pastor Deborah Ling founded Bless 'em Lord Ministries because she had a heart for the homeless. Having lived through three years of homelessness, she understands what they go through and has a program to help. The Lord has given her a vision for getting the homeless who want a hand up (not a handout) into transitional housing, getting them jobs to increase their income, and ultimately into permanent housing. She worked as a mentor with the homeless for about two years. Of those she mentored, two single moms and one couple moved on to permanent housing with their eight children.

mailto: pastordeb@blessemlord.org
Facebook:https://www.facebook.com/profile.php?id=100088664870517
LinkedIn: https://www.linkedin.com/in/bless-em-lord-30560225b/

Matt Love is the publisher of *Nestucca Spit Press* and the author of over 25 Oregon-themed books. He lives all around Oregon.

Marti MacGibbon, CADC-II Humorous Inspirational Speaker, nationally award-winning author, trauma expert and Addiction Certified Mental Health Professional, Gorski certified relapse-prevention specialist and member of the National Speakers Association. In the past, she hit rock bottom as a hard-core drug addict, was homeless, and was trafficked to Tokyo and held prisoner by Japanese organized crime. Her story of triumph is testimony to the power of the human spirit.

Facebook: www.facebook.com/MartiMac
LinkedIn: https://linkedin.com/in/martimacgibbon/
X: https://twitter.com/MartiMacGFB

Patricia McNair was raised in about 30 foster homes until age 12, then forced back with her bio mother. She has been abused since she was a baby on every level imaginable. She was drugged, kidnapped, and sold on the streets. As a nomad, she traveled for years and slept in her car. She is a four-time cancer survivor and has lived through two children being taken as she was a ward of the system. And that is just the physical side. "I will not be bitter but better! Love is the answer and the question."

mailto: connect@divineguidance.earth

Facebook: https://www.facebook.com/patricia.mcnair.988

YouTube: https://youtube.com/playlist?list=PL0DTaFbNAqSIdoH TJRE6b2Ov83hnAs1yW&si=GPGEditwfFg4zSDY

Brandy M. Miller is an award-winning creative strategist, international speaker, and author. She is also the visionary and co-producer of *Writing Reality TV Show*, which is available on YouTube. She is a member of the Board of Directors for *Path To Publishing* and the Program Development Director for the *Path To Connections* division.

mailto: 40daywriter@gmail.com.

Website: https://40daywriter.com

LinkedIn: https://www.linkedin.com/in/brandymmiller/

X: https://twitter.com/WriterBrandy

Instagram: https://instagram.com/DesignerBrandy

Zeina Navia is an eclectic soul who cares! She comes from a customer service/social service background. Xenia focuses on creative arts, sound frequencies, journalism, mentoring, and guiding one to heal their trauma.

Linda Forrester Pitocco is a retired law enforcement officer, a wife, mother of two, grandmother of four, writer, author, composer of faith-based music, devout Catholic, spiritual director, teacher, and artist.

mailto: xlynnsuelynn@yahoo.com

Sha'Kiera Star Randolph is a corporate trainer, speaker, and spoken word artist infused by her past of poverty and inspired by the promise of her future. She recently started sharing bits of her story in hopes of freeing herself from the impact of her upbringing and exposure to harsh inner city realities.

mailto:Info@kierastar.com

Website: http://kierastar.com/

Facebook: https://www.facebook.com/KieraStarSpoken

LinkedIn: https://www.linkedin.com/in/shakiera-star

Lonnee Rey dives headlong into the unknown. "The Professional Tumbleweed" has explored the darkest corners of the human psyche and mastered reinvention. Hosting transformational writing workshops for story-healers, she is the editor-in-chief of *Rattled Awake*, a unique-themed anthology series.

Website: https://www.officialrattledawake.com/

LinkedIn: https://www.linkedin.com/in/lonnee/

Aneesa Theron's personal philosophy is inspiring others and being a valuable contributor to society. She has a strong vision to contribute to the wealth of the economy creating value in organizations and people's lives. She leads with optimism, love, compassion, and a desire to live authentically Aneesa has been exposed to diverse roles during her professional career leading to self-leadership and mastery and a desire to make a positive social impact.

mailto: aneesatheron@gmail.com

Amrita Valen is a stay-at-home mom with two sons aged 14 and 15. She has worked in the hospitality industry, a five star hotel, and as content writer of deductive logic and reasoning in English test simulations for management entrance exam. She writes on any subject that sparks interests, such as food, religion, spirituality, mysticism, nature, children, emotion, and history.

mailto: amritavalan@gmail.com

Karin vonKrenner is a seasoned journalist and storyteller who passionately captures the essence of the human narrative through her words and lens. Her keen eye for detail and fusion of photography and writing unveil captivating global stories. Published in the *Middle East Journal* and other prestigious publications, Karin's work has been recognized through nominations for esteemed awards, solidifying her commitment to truth and establishing her as a respected and influential voice in journalism.

   mailto: kkrennerwriter@gmail.com

Mercedes Wright graduated from the University of Northern Colorado with a bachelor's in sociology and a minor in psychology. She is passionate about helping others reach their goals/vision by giving guidance and resources. She is currently working on becoming a certified trauma recovery coach. When she isn't helping others, she enjoys working on crafts or working outside.

Fred Young, a veteran, was unsheltered for five years in Indianapolis, Indiana. Drugs and alcohol took hold, forcing him on the street. His way back to sobriety and being clean led Fred to realize that mental health and anxiety were his deeper challenges. Fred has served veterans in many capacities and is now a peer specialist. His story, empathy, and caring show Fred's commit-ment to health, bettering himself, and serving others. Fred's faith had also been prominent in his healing journey.

   mailto: fredyoung1956@yahoo.com

Meet Our Media Partners

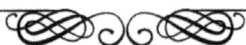

Eileen Bild is the CEO and Executive Producer at OTEL productions, ROKU Channel Developer, and Talk Show host for OTEL TALK. She is an author and internationally syndicated columnist for BizCatalyst360, *Life Coaching* magazine, *Women's Voice* magazine, and NSAEN. She is also a Breakthrough S.P.A.R.K. Coach.

    mailto: Info@EileenBild.com

    Website: https://www.oteluniverse.com/

    Website: www.corethinkingblueprint.com

Mark O'Brien is the founder principal of O'Brien Communications Group (obriencg.com), which he founded in 2004. He's also a lifelong writer, earning three Telly Awards and three U.S. International Film & Video Awards, and a columnist for BIZCATALYST 360°. You can see all his other published work on Amazon.

    mailto:mark@obriencg.com

    LinkedIn; https://www.linkedin.com/in/markobrien/

    Facebook: https://www.facebook.com/MarkNelsonOBrien

Heather Hansen O'Neill is a certified DiSC facilitator, TEDx Speaker (2x), author of *Find Your Fire* (Morgan James, 2011), *Teams On Fire!* (Rock Star Publishing House, 2013), and *Where's the Office?* (Authorhouse, 2021); Certified Corporate Success Coach, host of *Community Forum* TV show, guest expert on NBC, ABC, the CW, and FOX; columnist and feature article writer for several regional and national papers and magazines, co-host of *The Inspired Team Leader* radio show, producer of *Leading the Change: 21 Insights from the Experts*, founder of L-FOCUS (Leadership For Our Children's Ultimate Success), past Executive Director of the Bethel Chamber of Commerce, immediate past President of MPI WestField, Recommended MPI retreat facilitator and featured speaker at WEC, consultant on student and faculty engagement at the Ancell School of Business at Western CT State University, and creator and host of the popular *From Fear to Fire* podcast. Heather runs a successful business transforming lives and companies while expanding her mission of humanity.

mailto: heather@heatherhansenoneill.com

Website: https://heatherhansenoneill.com/

LinkedIn: https://www.linkedin.com/in/heatherhansenoneill/

Mark Reid hosts the Zen Sammich podcast. Previously, he was an English professor at Kanagawa University, Tokyo University of Science, and Ritsumeikan Asia Pacific University. He was also an attorney for 10 years, first as an Assistant District Attorney in New York state, and later worked in Securities Law for a large firm in Birmingham, Alabama. He now lives in the countryside of Japan and makes washi (traditional Japanese paper) for a living with his wife, Haruka. A graduate of the University of Alabama in political science and religion, with an MA from Florida State University in philosophy and ethics, and a JD from Syracuse University College of Law, he has a diversified background that through diligence and good fortune has taken him all over the world, including residential stints in Greece, England, and South Korea.

Website: http://zensammich.com/

LinkedIn: https://www.linkedin.com/in/zen-sammich/

Dr. Jo Anne White is an international multiple #1 bestselling, award-winning author, speaker, and trainer, Featured Contributor at BIZCATA-LYST 360°, and consultant recognized as a Goodwill Global Ambassador for civil and humanitarian work in education, entrepreneurship, coaching and women's issues. She was also named a Worldwide Branding Top Female Executive in Professional Coaching by Worldwide Who's Who. She's a certified life, spiritual and business coach, counselor and energy master teacher.

mailto: joanne@drjoannewhite.com

Christief in the City

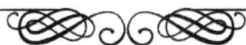

Christ in the City is a Catholic nonprofit dedicated to forming volunteers in their missionary identity and to learn how to know, love, and serve the poor. Young adults volunteer a year or two of their lives to live in community, undergo formation, and go to the streets to serve the chronically homeless. The missionaries strive to know, love, and serve the poor through a consistent presence and friendship on the streets, and through this, hope that the poor see their dignity. The missionaries train over a thousand volunteers of all ages every year to join them at a weekly meal where the greater community is invited into friendship with the poor.

More info on *Christ in the City* can be found at www.christinthecity.org.

www.ingramcontent.com/pod-product-compliance
Lightning Source LLC
Chambersburg PA
CBHW070055030426
42335CB00016B/1897